The Beauty Play Book

The Beauty Play Book

The Beauty Play Book

70 practical practices to help improve your beauty habits

by

Nicole Stromberg- The Hair Coach

Copyright © 2019 by Alexandria Nicole Stromberg

Copyright © 2019 Cover Art by Robert D. Stromberg

All Rights Reserved

ISBN 13: 9781091485075

Alexandria Nicole Stromberg-The Beauty Play Book-70 Practical Practices To Help Improve Your Beauty Habits

<u>Acknowledgements</u>

Praise Be To God for ALL Things. To my clients, I dedicate this book to you. Thank you for entrusting me with your hair and for the relationships we have developed over the years.

To all my Cosmetology Colleagues what an honor it has been to serve with you in this industry for all these years. I am forever grateful to you all for including me in your professional lives. It has definitely been an adventure!

To my Cosmetology Students past and present, this book is for you! Let this book be a true example to you of what you can accomplish if you set your mind to the task.

I would also like to thank my husband, Rob. For putting up with me and all the things I try my hand at, for his tireless labor of love in helping bring this vision to life. You are my biggest cheerleader and I am forever grateful for you and for everything you do for our family. To my sons, Alex and Keagan, thank you for being the best gift God has given me. And to my mother-in-law, Pat, you're and amazing person and I can't thank you enough for your support. Thanks for always listening to my wild ideas and for keeping me grounded. Special shout out to my photographer Jim Hopper and to each and every person whose had a hand in making this book a success. I am forever grateful.

Much love to you all,

Nicole

<u>Introduction</u>

In these pages you will find classic beauty tips and instruction from the *play book* of an expert Cosmetologist. Some of the beauty tips may remind you of things you already know and then again you may be reading it for the first time. I like to refer to them as classics that never die. No matter the season or stage you are in, allow this book to educate, guide and challenge you to take better care of you and your beauty needs. The Beauty Play Book offers you 70 practical practices to help improve your beauty habits created with the client in mind.

Congratulations! You have already taken the first step to learning more helpful suggestions to enhancing your beauty habits. So sit back, relax, take notes, and enjoy this inspiring book. Feel free to share it with others and use it as a reference for many years to come. Please know that all suggestions and recommendations have been tried and are deemed as true from the many years I have stood behind the chair and made these very suggestions to my clients and students.

Read on. You won't be disappointed.

Endorsements

"Madame Boss Nicole is my sister from another mister. She is gifted in what she does and has helped me overcome a personal insecurity that I have dealt with for some time now concerning my hair. I think you are the bomb.com and I am thankful for what you have done for me as my hairdresser and friend. "

> --Andrea "Bug" Brown, High School Hall of Fame, Community Leader, Client

"Nicole has been my hairdresser since 1998. Becoming her client was a blessing in more ways than one. First, she is a Christian who loves the Lord. Second, she cares about my spiritual, physical, and mental health as well as the health of my hair and external being. Last, but certainly not least; I love and trust her so much that she has been the only hairdresser for my daughters who have been visiting Nicole since the age of 5. My daughters are now 16 and 10. She has not only cared for their hair but has treated them as if they are her own by giving motherly advice and participating in girl conversations.

Nicole has kept my daughters' and my hair healthy and beautiful from the inside out and teaches us that what we put in our bodies is a reflection of the health of our hair and skin. Nicole is THE best and I am blessed to be her friend and client. She keeps me beautiful externally and internally. Her level of professionalism and chairside manner surpasses all others."

> --Stephanie Williams, Client

"Mrs. Nicole has taught me MANY things since becoming my instructor. One thing that will always stand out to me is she told me I was and Overcomer. Not really knowing the depth of what that actually meant she has SHOWN me through all the things I have gone through in my life (being a single mother, not having a mother, mental illness, sickness and other life challenges). She has shown me that I WILL overcome! As cheesy as it sounds, you have been the most support I've EVER had since my grandmother passed away some years ago."

> --Shareka "Bodacious Beauty" Miller, Student

"I met Nicole Stromberg in 2001. I saw the results of my neighbors' hair and had to know who was doing her hair! I made my first appointment the next day and I have been with Nicole ever since. She is all about healthy hair and that's what I love the most. My hair is healthy, and always looks amazing. My hair has never looked or felt as good as it does under Nicole's care. "I tell her all the time, she has blessed hands and can never retire!"

--Trina Black, Client

"I am thankful for everything Mrs. Nicole has done for me. She is an amazing person. I positively wouldn't have been able to pass my cosmetology exam without her confidence in me and the knowledge she shared while I was in school. I love her dearly."

-Sara L. Pike, Former Student

Contents

The Hair Practices

The Skin Care And Cosmetic Practice

Nicole-

The Hair Coach.

Teaching the Beauty

Consumer.

The Beauty Play #1

Taking Time Out

The Beauty Play By Play:

Taking time for yourself is probably the hardest thing you are faced with in today's time. As hard as you work and as committed as you are to the day-to-day responsibilities, there is not enough time in the day for much of anything else, especially if you have family and/or a demanding career. Those two things alone or combined are usually the determining factors as to how your day goes and what you have time to do for yourself.

Beauty rest is important. You-must-rest! You need to get as much rest as you can so you will be able to handle the demands in your life. When you rest, you will notice the circles under your eyes start to diminish. You will notice that your skin looks rested. You don't look as worn out as you were. You will notice you have a little bit more clarity and direction for the day. Your mood is better and you're not as overwhelmed or anxious as before. I know when I get enough rest I feel like I can conquer the world. After all, you are to be more than a conqueror right?

Taking time out for yourself can be a hobby like shopping, reading, meditating, having quiet time, working out, going to get your hair or nails done, going to get a massage, spending time with family and friends. It's doing something other than your normal routine.

Whatever you do outside of the hustle of life, do it in the name of you! I'm sure you deserve it.

The Beauty Practice:

Just like you commit to so many other things for so many other people, learn to commit to something for yourself. I give you permission to be just a little selfish for a few minutes.

Try going to bed earlier than your normal time, even if it's only 30 minutes earlier. This will at least help get your mind to slow down and begin to relax.

Think about an activity you did years ago. Something that doesn't make you feel like another task, but something you did before you became so busy. Try to do that special thing that was positive, relaxing and brought you joy.

BE WHO YOU ARE, NOT WHO THE WORLD WANTS YOU TO BE.

-COCO CHANEL-

The Beauty Play #2

You Are What You Eat

The Beauty Play by Play:

This is one of the most challenging things to do in today's microwave and fast food society. When I ask my clients about what they eat, they usually give me the rundown of what they have had for the day.

Like most, my clients are always on the go and so their eating habits vary. But I always know the ones that take the time to cook their own meals and I know which ones don't take the time to prepare home cooked meals.

When I ask the questions: What do you eat? What do you like to cook? When was the last time you cooked? I get responses and reactions that imply eating healthy is expensive. My personal favorite: I skip meals and don't drink water. On the other hand, I do have those clients that actually plan their meals and keep a balanced diet. You have to remember that what you put in your body comes out through your pores (skin), your hair and nails. When your body is unhealthy on the inside, it will be the same on the outside. You really are what you eat, so be mindful how you treat your body and pay attention to what you put into your body.

It is a fact that other than your medical professional, your hairdresser will be able to detect when you have changed things within your diet; most of the time your hair and skin will become extremely dry or extremely oily because of what you are ingesting into your body. You may experience a lot of shedding from your hair, more than the normal 80-100 strands shed per day. Pay attention to your hair, nails and your skin: they will tell you what you need to know for your body. Believe it or not, your hairdresser becomes a vital part in your personal appearance. I have found that most clients consult the stylist before they consult with any other professional. They wait to see what the stylist recommends and then they may follow through with the recommendation of that person.

The Beauty Practice:

Pay attention to what your hair and body is saying to you.

Try not to skip meals and by all means make sure you are drinking plenty of water.

Make healthier eating choices.

When you go to restaurants, choose from the healthier side of the menu.

The Beauty Play #3

Drink More Water

The Beauty Play by Play:

We need water to help keep our bodies hydrated inside and out. Wouldn't you agree? Water is the most essential part of our health. Water is great for our hair, skin and nail growth structure.

I have seen many clients come to the salon and talk about how dry their hair or their skin is and then they begin to self-diagnosis themselves with different skin disorders because they don't drink enough water. Water is such an important component to our body. When it comes to our hair and skin water seems to be overlooked as a key component to health of it. Let me share with you 10 benefits of water for your crown of glory that I have learned over the years:

1. Water helps rid the toxins out of your body and it helps to get rid of unwanted scalp and skin conditions.
2. Water helps to hydrate and transform dull, lifeless dry hair and skin.
3. Water helps promote hair growth and weight loss all at the same time.
4. Water acts as a natural neutralizer. It helps to maintain the PH balance of the body, hair and skin.
5. Drinking one glass of water when you wake up will help jumpstart your metabolism.

6. A cool water rinse after conditioner helps add a great shine to the hair. It also seals the hair cuticle and helps calm down the frizzes, allowing each strand of hair to be smooth.
7. Water helps soften the skin.
8. Alkaline water tastes better than regular tap water, spring or purified water.
9. Water helps to energize your body and does the same for your skin, hair and nails.
10. Water is usually one of the first five ingredients in your hair and skin products.

The Beauty Practice:

Drink your recommend amount of water a day per your weight. To help drink 1 glass of water at the top of every hour, set a reminder in your phone to help you remember to drink more water.

Drink that first glass of water within the first hour of being awake.

Replace your favorite beverage with water. Sorry, no cheating. No adding any flavored packets to your water either. You can add fresh or frozen fruits or vegetables to your water, such as strawberries, watermelon, cucumber, lemon or limes. This makes for a refreshing drink and it adds flavor to the water naturally.

The Beauty Play #4

Hair Vitamins

The Beauty Play by Play:

For years I was against using Hair Vitamins. I believed that there was no need for them. I have always been a pretty healthy eater and active most of my life, so I didn't see the benefits of using hair vitamins until now.

As I have said earlier, in this microwave and fast food society, we are always in a hurry or on a time schedule for something or someone. It wasn't until recently that I even considered this type of vitamin. One of my new clients asked me if I could recommend any hair vitamins to her because of the damaged condition her hair was in during her appointment with me. I proceeded to tell her my beliefs on hair vitamins, that if she would just eat healthy and drink water and exercise she would be helping her hair get back to a healthy state and she would not need any hair vitamins. She agreed and said she is trying to eat better and walk when she can, but in the mean time she wanted to incorporate hair vitamins. I shared with her that the company I get my vitamins from just released their hair, skin & nail vitamins. I offered to order her the hair vitamins and she could judge for herself if they would work for her or not.

I ordered her first 30 day supply, and before the end of her first 30 day, we both noticed a difference in her hair. I still wasn't convinced so she ordered a second bottle. After 60 days she had new growth in her troubled spots on her head. She noticed her nails were growing and she always had problems growing her nails. I began my research about these vitamins and found these vitamins, minerals and herbal supplements were formulated to help improve hair growth, strengthen follicles and help promote healthy hair and skin. The vitamins help maintain the care of the hair, nail and skin structure. This began to get my attention.

My clients commitment to taking the supplements showed me that they were an added bonus to my work and we go hand in hand. The fantastic results she is getting allowed me to share with my other clients that hair vitamins are not so bad after all. They actually help promote the health of the hair that we lose from poor diet, medications, and from the weather.

Since I have witnessed the change in my clients hair, I have become a believer in these particular company's hair, skin and nail vitamins. I do know not if all of them work for everyone, and I make sure I encourage my clients to seek their doctor's approval on any type of vitamins or medications they may take. I can suggest, but it's still up to the person to find out what's best for them. Everyone's systems may react differently to vitamins based on their medical history.

The Beauty Practice:

Consult with your healthcare provider before you try hair, nail or skin vitamins, they may recommend a particular brand to you. Make sure you are not just taking any kind. Make sure your vitamins are quality and are backed by a medical board or team.

Drink plenty of water with all vitamins.

Give them time to work (I recommend 90 days).

The Beauty Play #5

Choose Properly

The Beauty Play by Play:

If I had a dollar for every time I heard a client, consumer or my beauty school students talk about the shampoo and conditioner they just randomly choose to *just* cleanse and condition their hair, I would be pretty wealthy! This is one of the most important decisions to start with, to get great results for the hair and scalp.

I agree there are a lot of choices out on the market, but we have to take the time in choosing the right one for your particular needs.

Consider these three things I share with my clients:

1. Shampoo is to help cleanse the hair and scalp and to remove all impurities. It also helps treat a specific need for your hair. It could be to strengthen the hair or to clarify the hair. Depending on if your hair is chemically treated hair, blonde or natural hair.

2. Conditioners are an aide after the hair has been shampooed and properly cleansed. It is to deposit what the shampoo removed from the hair. For example, if the hair was really dry, you would use a moisturizing conditioner to condition the hair.

3. Shampoo's ultimate job is to remove all dirt, debris and oil from the hair and conditioner puts back into the hair what was removed from the shampoo.

Here is another one of my favorite examples for individuals to truly understand what I actually mean: Together shampoo and conditioner go hand in hand, like soap is to our body and water is to rinse it away. That always seems to make the light bulb go off in their heads and actually put it all in context. It's a really good analogy it helps people understand where I am coming from.

The Beauty Practice:

Seek professionals first. Allow them to prescribe the correct shampoo and conditioner for your hair type. When this is done, you will notice an improvement in your hair.

Become a label reader. Always read the label for your shampoos and conditioners. Make sure you are getting more than a bottle of water in the brands you choose.

Purchase only from salons or your stylist. Try the smaller size bottles before you invest in the larger bottles.

The Beauty Play #6

You Get What You Pay For

The Beauty Play by Play:

In all the years I have been a hairdresser there has been a consistent response to getting clients to purchase hair products from hair stylists. Most clients think the products we suggest for them to take home are WAY TOO EXPENSIVE! They look at the size of bottle and hear the price and immediately they think it is highway robbery in some cases. The truth of the matter is when you switch to the professional hair products, you use less than you would use from the products you purchase at the local grocery or retail store.

There is a BIG difference in using the grocery store brand than using the high end brand. The professional products are highly concentrated, which means you use less than you would with the off brand products. This is the first savings to using these products that are specifically chosen by the stylist for your particular hair care needs. You should also consider using the products your stylist suggests so they know what is being used on the hair in case a problem or issue arises in your hair and scalp. As a cosmetologist there is nothing more aggravating than when problems arise and clients are not using the correct products recommended by the stylist. It's so much easier to help you in the problems with the hair if you are using professional recommended products for your specific hair. If you trust the person to perform a hair service on your hair, trust them with their recommendations too. You won't regret paying a little more for what is going to give you the best care for your hair. It's that old saying: you get what you pay for! If you want just "ok" hair, you will buy "ok" products. If you want that hair to look and feel like it does after you leave the hair salon, then go ahead and purchase those amazing products that have been made with you in mind. Your hair will thank you.

The Beauty Practice:

Trust the educated stylist to assist you with your high end products.

The education your stylist can provide is beneficial in advising you as to what products you need to purchase. They will be able to share with you some tips on how and why this is the product that will work best for your hair.

You don't have to buy the big bottles first. Ask the stylist for a sample of the products they are recommending. Most of the time they will be able to give you a sample. If it is a product they just used, you will get to experience the benefits right then, and that will help you in your decision to purchase or not to purchase those particular products.

The Beauty Play #7

Cutting Cost

The Beauty Play by Play:

Be careful what you watch and try to do from YouTube and other social media platforms. My colleagues and I have many conversations about the people who come into the salon to get us to fix what they tried to do from the crash course from YouTube University (as we call it). It makes it very difficult to have to fix a mess that was created by you and your big ideas. I know it seems pretty easy from the video clips you watch, but that's not always the case when you begin the service yourself. Your arms get tired and your back begins to hurt. Products (color especially) are all over your bathroom. It starts to become a mess. Not to mention you're not as proficient or as quick as the stylist would be in getting the product applied. You take the risk of becoming the spotted leopard. Don't get me wrong. I know there are many things we all learn from YouTube. It's helpful in many ways and I know this picture I have painted here does not apply to everyone. But when it comes to doing highlights, color, relaxers, and straighteners, please leave that to the trained professionals. These are services that just should not be done at home. In many cases, I know you try to do it to cut cost. Haven't you learned that it will cost you more to correct what you have attempted than just simply going to the salon? You owe it to yourself to be pampered. You will thank me later. This choice will be worth the investment and health of your hair.

The Beauty Practice:

Take time for yourself (see The Beauty Play #1)! Schedule your appointment with a qualified stylist in your area.

Check their social media page to see what they offer and what they may charge.

Check the reviews of the salon and the stylist to see if it will be a good fit for you.

If it is a service that is pricey you may want to start saving. Therefore, when you go to your appointment with the stylist you won't feel like it's so taxing on your pockets. My clients make me a part of their budget. This helps them and it helps the stylist. If only all clients could do this.

INVEST IN YOUR HAIR;

IT IS THE ONLY CROWN YOU WILL NEVER TAKE OFF!

The Beauty Play #8

The Right Stylist

The Beauty Play by Play:

There are many people who don't understand the importance of choosing a stylist. It is so important because your hairdresser becomes one of the most important people in your life. You want to take the time to meet the right stylist for that reason alone, not to mention the right stylist can be with you through many important events in your life like: your first haircut and through your prom hair styles. Beyond prom, your faithful stylist can be with you through the biggest days of your life: your high school or college graduation, your wedding day, your first child, the loss of a love one, or maybe even a divorce. Whatever the season may be in your life, a devoted stylist will be right there with you. A great example of this is my client that has been with me since the age of 12 and now she is in her early 30's. Recently I helped another client of 10 years prepare for her father's funeral. There are many more reasons why I suggest finding that special hairdresser; we help you look your best when you may not feel your best.

There are many stylists who are trained and qualified with passion and integrity for the beauty industry. Choosing a stylist should be like an investment into your life. You are choosing someone who can give you a great haircut or color and should also be able to give you some sound advice. Someone you will end up spending quite a bit of time with. Someone who will tell you the truth as to what is going to look good on you. Think of it as a return on investment (ROI). You are investing in the hairdresser who is now investing their skill and talents in you. As stylists, we are put in a unique position to help those in need for more than just your hair.

It's simple, you invest in us and we invest in you, our time, skills and ability to give you the desired look you want to achieve, a relationship, a friendship and many times a lasting partnership.

The Beauty Practice:

If you currently do not have a stylist, ask around and get recommendations from people you know and trust, especially if you have moved to a new city or state.

Hairdressers are visual people. Taking pictures of haircuts, the desired hair color or style helps the stylist perform a more efficient and accurate service for you, leaving you happy and pleased with what you desired.

Don't wait long periods of time to rebook with your stylist. Good stylists book up pretty quickly, go ahead and schedule your appointment before you leave the salon. Then set a reminder in your phone of the appointment you just made. This helps you to schedule your time in advance as well as the stylist who sets aside that particular time in their appointment book just for you! This helps with your future visits to the salon.

The Beauty Play #9

Shampooing Etiquette

The Beauty Play by Play:

Were you aware that there is a proper way to shampoo your hair? Well there is. One of the reasons you have so many tangles in the hair after you shampoo is due to the improper scrubbing and scratching of the hair. Everyone loves a good shampoo, and we tend to think more scratching of the nails on the scalp makes it a better experience and makes the hair cleaner. This is not the case. The main reason we shampoo the hair is to get rid of the oils, sweat, make-up, product build-up and grime. But in all actuality, we should be concerned about our scalp and the proper care for it. How we scrub the scalp when shampooing the hair is very important. Scratching the scalp with our nails is an improper method and also a myth. It's all in the pads of your fingertips!

When nails are used during the lathering, they cut the hair and cause premature shedding. It also roughens the hair and makes it harder to comb out, even with use of conditioners after the shampoo. You also become more susceptible to injury to the scalp. Using your natural nails can and will leave you with irritations, cuts and scrapes to the scalp.

Use shampooing etiquette, when shampooing your hair. Make sure your fingertips go underneath the hair onto the scalp while applying pressure as you are manipulating and stimulating the scalp while cleansing. This serves to be a much more effective technique and it still cleans the hair and scalp.

I will admit using the cushions of your fingertips does take some time to get used to doing and the feel is a little different. As you get comfortable using the pressure from your fingers, you will begin to see a difference in the way you shampoo the hair. The feel of shampooing with the balls of your fingertips becomes more preferred over those hard nails. You will also have fewer tangles when you comb your hair out afterwards.

The Beauty Practice:

Just try it before you automatically decide against it; your scalp will thank you!

Practice using the cushions of your fingertips verses your nails when shampooing your hair.

You may need to shampoo the hair a few seconds longer than usual and make sure you apply pressure to your shampooing with your new technique.

The Beauty Play #10

Product Lines Matter

The Beauty Play by Play:

One important discovery I had early in my career as a cosmetologist was to use the same product line on my clients hair. When I used a shampoo from Brand X, I made sure I used the same conditioner from Brand X.

This discovery became overwhelming to me when I realized the amount of products I was using at the shampoo bowl. My clients would ask me on their follow up appointment, "What did you use in my hair?" "When, I would ask?" Sometimes my clients could pinpoint exactly when, and at other times they could not. This made it hard on me to give them the correct answer. I knew then something had to change.

Once I began to listen to what they were asking me, I quickly found that I was not always using the same product line during their service. I would use a little bit of this and a little bit of that. Although, I would choose based on the need of the clients hair; I just wouldn't use the same product line throughout the process. Then one day a faithful client came into the salon with a lot of shedding going on with her hair. She was a weekly patron so she did not shampoo her hair on her own; she left her hair in my hands. It was that day when I realized that I could not tell her what I used in her hair because I always mixed my product lines together. I would use Product line A with Brand X. I was good at being a "Mixologist" of different products until this occurrence happened to me.

I was caught by surprise with the results of my clients hair and from that day I realized it's not always beneficial to mix product lines. It is easier to use one complete line on a person than to use several. This way it helps you to identify any problems or challenges that may happen along the way. Now I can pinpoint exactly what I use on a person's hair from beginning to end. I minimized my product selections and began using the products according to the manufacturer's directions.

Product lines are made to use together. They are formulated per the brand line, which means, the manufacturing company knows what works well when combined with their other products. This information assists the stylist and the consumer when choosing the products best suited for the needs of their hair.

The Beauty Practice:

Most companies now have a variety of selections to choose from their product lines for all your hair care needs.

Stop mixing the brands in case a problem with your hair does arise. This will help you gather information on what works for your hair and what doesn't work, and maybe steer clear of a particular hair care line you are using.

Try the smaller bottles first before you invest in bigger bottles for long term use.

The Beauty Play #11

The Switch

The Beauty Play by Play:

It's a good idea to switch your products. I suggest to my clients who maintain their hair at home to change their shampoo and conditioners once a month. I believe this gives the hair a jumpstart and allows the hair to get other nutrients that may be missing from the normal products they use. You can use a totally different line from the start! Just keep it all together. Let me also advise you not to pick a product line because it smells good. It is nice to use good smelling products, but you have to make sure that the fragrance that lures you to purchase it actually has some benefits other than the scent.

The Beauty Practice:

When you use products for moisture, then choose an alternate line for strength.

Choose a line that contains tea tree oil because it helps stimulate the blood flow to the scalp.

Whatever line you choose, make sure you use the products that work together.

The Beauty Play #12

Old School Method

The Beauty Play by Play:

As a child, one of my favorite activities before I went to bed was to brush my hair 100 strokes because I thought it would make my hair grow long. Fast forward to becoming a hairdresser and finding out the science behind this myth; I have learned that brushing the hair actually helps to stimulate the scalp and increase circulation. It also helps to relax a tight scalp that can occur from a busy day. Brushing the hair does encourage the oil glands to wake up and produce more nutrients to the scalp and hair.

Might I also suggest, if your hair is naturally oily, you may want to brush with fewer strokes. Whatever your hair type may be, dry, average, or oily, I still recommend brushing your hair at night, it is extremely relaxing.

The Beauty Practice:

Brushing the hair at night has additional benefits. It helps you get into a calm and restful with each stroke.

You can add some good *Soaking Music* to this activity to really help you get prepared for a restful night.

Choose a paddle or cushion brush to brush your hair. This kind of brush is a must have because the balls on the tips of the brush make it a soothing experience.

The Beauty Play #13

Secrets of a Satin Pillowcase

The Beauty Play by Play:

For years, I have recommended to women to sleep on satin pillowcases to help keep their hairstyles. Many years have passed and I am still recommending the same satin pillowcases, now for different reasons. The satin cases not only keep the hairstyle, you don't wake up with as much "bedhead" as with a cotton pillowcase. They help keep and maintain the moisture and sheen in the hair and do not cause you to sweat like cotton does. Cotton tends to make the hair dry and dull, eventually causing unwanted hair troubles later. Satin pillowcases help to stop the hair from breakage and excessive shedding. Sleeping on this particular material eliminates the granny caps and doo-rags women wear at night to preserve our hairstyles. One more reason is the person next to you at night doesn't have to see you with the bonnet on. It is certainly not very romantic to say the least. If you are having your "personal summers" (hot-flashes), not wearing a bonnet helps to allow your head to breathe and not hold all that extra heat. In my opinion, satin pillowcases are much softer and cooler when you lay on them than the plain old cotton pillowcases.

I am so serious about sleeping on a satin pillowcase I take my personal one with me when I travel. I can't afford to let that average pillowcase affect my hair. Plus, I don't want to have to do any more work to my hair than necessary.

The Beauty Practice:

Purchase your satin pillowcase today! You can find them at the local retail stores or you can order them online. You will be glad you did.

Order/purchase more than one pillowcase. This way when you have to wash one, you can replace it with a clean one. I normally air dry mine, but check the manufacturer's directions for preferred maintenance.

If you normally wear a bonnet, pay close attention to how the satin pillowcase makes you feel and how your hairstyle will stay intact. I believe you will agree with me and say, the satin pillowcase works better than the bonnet.

The Beauty Play #14

The Brush Cleanse

The Beauty Play by Play:

I can remember reminding my clients to clean their hair brushes after getting their hair done. To my surprise this was not something they were accustomed to doing. Most of my clients looked at me as if I had just spoken another language to them. I have learned that cleansing your hair tools is not at the top of the priority list for a lot of people. Many of my clients told me that they just didn't think about cleaning their hair brushes. They just keep on using them. So now I remind them at their hair appointment to make sure they use clean combs and brushes with their clean hairdo. It's important to have clean hair and scalp. So why not take it a step further and clean your combs and brushes!

Believe it or not, I did run across a client who told me she would always throw away her hair brushes and buy new ones. She said, "I'm just that lazy and I don't like cleaning my brushes anyway." Whatever your choice is, let me enlighten you to the importance of cleaning your brushes… but first let me ask you a few questions:

1. Who wants to use dirty brushes on clean hair?
2. What's the point of cleaning your hair if you don't clean your tools?
3. If you developed scalp irritation how would you know when you may have gotten it, if you're not in the habit of cleaning your combs and brushes?

Now the important part:

Taking just a few minutes after cleansing your hair to wash your brushes can help get rid of debris, dandruff and unwanted bacteria from the scalp.

When you cleanse your brushes, it can also help to stop spreading any type of odor or excess oil that may have accumulated in your brushes. It's very unhealthy for the scalp and could cause unwanted issues to the hair. There is nothing more irritating, embarrassing and noticeable than dandruff or dead skin falling from the scalp and resting on the shoulders of your clothes. These two issues can be prevented if you clean your brushes, combs, picks, etc. Dandruff can be contagious. That's why, I can't stress enough what cleaning those hair tools can do for the hair and scalp.

Here is what I do:

I recommend having several hair brushes, maybe even various choices of brush, and rotate them (dirty for clean). This way you don't feel like you are constantly cleaning brushes. Typically, I shampoo my hair once a week. Depending on how often you shampoo your hair, will determine how often you will clean your combs and brushes. Once you get in a habit of rotating and cleaning your brushes and combs, it won't feel time consuming.

The Beauty Practice:

Start now! Go and gather up all your combs, brushes and whatever else you may use for styling your hair and go wash them.

You can use your shampoo or you can purchase brush cleaner for your utensils. It's up to you.

Get in the habit of cleaning your tools often!

The Beauty Play #15

Ready, Set, Curl!

The Beauty Play by Play:

Did you know there is an art to curling hair? It doesn't matter if it is curled with a curling iron, flat iron, and wand or by sitting under the hooded dryer with rollers (a.k.a. curlers). When you style the hair, it is considered a style that does not have any permanent change to the hair; which means, the bonds in the hair have only been temporarily changed. These particular hair styles will not last long. Depending on the style, the weather, and the person wearing the style, you might not get through the night with your hairstyle.

When you use heated styling tools such as a curling iron or flat iron, you want to make sure that after you make the curl in the hair you "set" the curl to allow the curl to stay in the pattern that you desire. Make sure to incorporate good thermal-heat products on the hair to aid in your desired look.This helps to tell the hair what you want it to do. This works well for women with long hair. The weight of long hair pulls the curl down and doesn't allow the curl to stay. It ends up being more like a wave than a curl. Cooling the hair for all lengths makes a difference, especially on shoulder length or longer hair.

If you are still in the habit of getting rolled up and set with rollers (curlers) under the dryer, the same rule still applies. Have you ever paid attention to the hooded dryer? You sit under the dryer until the time runs out and the dryer begins to cool. It's the cooling that helps to keep the curls set in by the rollers and the heat, which dries the hair. Even with your roller-sets coming out from under the dryer, you should wait 2-3 minutes before you begin to remove the rollers out of the hair and begin to style the hair to the desired look.

The benefits of this curling method are as follows:

1. Letting the set cool makes the curls more firm and helps it last longer.
2. It helps with the memory of what you want the hair to do. You tell it what to do and it does just that.
3. This set is temporary and will only last for a few days before you have to shampoo and reset or re-curl the hair all over again.

The Beauty Practice:

When curling the hair with your hot tools, hold each curl until the hair is cooled off. If you are going to set your entire head, you may want to use clips or bobby pins to hold the curls in place.

Use styling products to help you achieve and save your temporary hairstyle.

Thermal sets are temporary.

NO MATTER WHO YOU ARE NO MATTER WHERE YOU COME FROM YOU ARE BEAUTIFUL.

-Michelle Obama

The Beauty Play #16

Read the Labels

The Beauty Play by Play:

It is common at any given time to read the labels on the back of the foods we eat: can goods, frozen items or even the meat in the meat department. We get very particular in percentages that are in our meats (80% lean 20% fat) when picking which hamburger we want to purchase. We make sure to see how many calories are in certain foods, especially our sweet treat we like to eat. So I pose the question: Why don't we do that for hair products we purchase?

Recently, I purchased a product from my favorite hair care company, and I didn't hesitate once on price. I knew what I was getting was quality. I have not had a bad product from this company. I purchased the merchandise, complimented the sales clerk about the packaging and just went on and on about the total look of the product. I took my purchase home and the very next day I shampooed and conditioned with my new shampoo and conditioner. I dried and styled my hair as usual. I did notice that around my hairline my hair was a little bit drier than normal, but I shrugged it off and went about my day. Well, as the day progressed, my scalp went from an itch to a burn. My scalp itched so bad it kept me up at night for a week before I figured out what was wrong with my scalp. I was having an allergic reaction to my new product I just purchased! My scalp became inflamed and blisters began to form. It was an awful experience!

I ended up going back to my other brand I was using and I began to feel immediate relief. My scalp was still sore to the touch and I couldn't tolerate brushing, but soon I began to feel the burn simmer down. I went back to my new products I purchased and read the labels. Just like I taught you in Play #10 and Play #12. I failed at reading the ingredients on the very back of the bottle. And when I finally read the labels I realized there was an ingredient in the product that my body is sensitive to internally. My eyes were big as golf balls when I discovered this ingredient. I was glad to know I found the culprit, and now I had to suffer from not doing the one thing we all should do, read the labels! We can save ourselves a lot of time, money and discomfort.

The Beauty Practice:

READ THE PRODUCT LABELS on the front and back of the items you intend to purchase. It will save you from the itch and the burn!

The Beauty Play #17

Stress is No Joke

The Beauty Play by Play:

Stress tends to bring on so many problems with our bodies that we tend to forget what it does to the hair. Stress is one of the causes that does affect your hair and causes it to shed or come completely out.

Here are a few examples of what stress can look like. For starters, not allowing yourself to get the necessary sleep to replenish the body comes from stress. Developing dark circles and bags under your eyes is another sign. Your hair suffers by getting dry and limp. Possible hair thinning, which can lead to Alopecia Areata. Which is when the hair can come out in patches; it could come out in small or larger areas of the head.

I don't like telling my clients who are already stressed out that their stress is affecting their hair but I have to be the bearer of bad news at times. It is the job of the caring Professional Hairdresser to tell you how your stress is affecting your hair just like the rest of your body and your overall health. Stress is no joke and the sooner you realize what's going on, the sooner you can come up with a plan to bring your stress level down. Stress has been known to take people out of this world by heart attacks and strokes. I know this seems severe since we are just talking about hair. Just know it is all possible. Stress does not go away by ignoring the symptoms and problems. Take your stress level seriously and get some relief.

The Beauty Practice:

Pay attention to your stress level.

Get a game plan together to help bring down or even eliminate your stress. Get some relief.

When it comes to your hair being affected by your stress, let your hairdresser know what's going on so they will know how to treat the hair accordingly.

By all means contact your Family Physician so they know what's going on with you so they can help assist you in the matter as well.

We only get one shot at this thing called life. Do your best to eliminate stress!

The Beauty Play #18

K.I.S.S

The Beauty Play by Play:

It amazes me that after all these years and all the research that has been done, we still ask the question whether it is a good idea to use products that contain the shampoo and conditioner all in one (2-in-1). Now they have added the body soap inside with the shampoo and conditioner (3-in-1). I know that most of the time this is a good marketing tool to use for men. It is also a good marketing tool to save on time when shampooing your hair. We think let's "kill two birds with one stone," so to speak. When in all actuality this method does not work effectively. For each product in the bottle it either dilutes each other or your hair does not get the right amount of shampoo or conditioner needed to cleanse or condition the hair well. If you add body soap into the mix, the 3-in-1, in my opinion, you are not likely to get the conditioning benefits your hair needs. You are more likely to get the fragrance if anything.

Although the idea of all the product ingredients being in one bottle sounds convenient and time saving, it's not. In the long run, using these 2-in-1 and/or 3-in-1 products will eventually cause the hair to miss out on proper cleansing and nutrients needed for your hair type. Your hair may become extremely dehydrated and brittle from too much shampoo and not enough conditioner. Or it could to be extremely oily from the hair not being properly cleansed and the conditioner could add to the oils and dirt that's already in the hair. If you throw the body soap into the mix, no telling what the hair is going to feel like after using it wet or dry.

My professional advice to you is to K.I.S.S "Keep It Separate Sweetie!"

The Beauty Practice:

Keep your shampoo, conditioner, and your body soap separate.

Purchase these products for your hair type and not for the convenience of the "All-In-One."

Take time out to educate yourself on what is going to be beneficial for your hair texture, hair type and for your overall hair needs.

The Beauty Play #19

Be Delicate to the Damaged

The Beauty Play By Play:

In my opinion, there is nothing worse than having damaged hair. It doesn't matter how much you condition it. No matter how much you try to do to the hair, the best thing is to just cut it off and start all over. Well, ok. You don't have to be that drastic, but it is the sure way to bring your hair back to a healthy state.

Your damaged hair is in a very dry, fragile, and sensitive condition. It is important to be delicate to the damaged. I recommend that you seek the professional. Make an appointment with your hairdresser and allow them to assess the situation and determine what is going to be best for your hair. You may have to prolong getting your chemical services until your hair becomes healthy again. You may need a series of deep conditionings that contain moisture, strength (protein) or certain oils. Another suggestion I would give is to get your hair cut or trimmed. Cutting and/or trimming the hair can help take off some of the damaged hair and help put your hair on the road to recovery. Be patient and treat the damaged hair delicately with tender loving care.

The Beauty Practice:

<u>Drastic Measure</u>- Cut all the damaged hair off and start all over.

Seek the professional for an assessment of what type of treatments your hair may need.

Prolong all chemical services until your hair is able to handle them.

The Beauty Play #20

Cocktails for the Hair

The Beauty Play by Play:

Before you go thinking about your favorite beverage and getting all thirsty, let me share with you what I mean exactly. Just like you would any of your favorite beverages, you can do the same for your hair treatments. It's pretty much the same fun exciting concept. In this case you won't be tasting; you will be feeling the hair to determine if you are going to like your concoction. You can mix a little bit of this and a little bit of that to get the achieved taste. In your hair's case it's going to be the achieved balance of products for a specific purpose for the health of the hair.

Many product manufacturers have several different products that can be used together even though they are in two or three separate bottles. You can add them together and use them as your hair treatments. Products are made to be universal within their own brand and you can be your own chemist or mixologist. You know your hair better than anyone, so giving yourself treatments at home can help you maintain what your stylist has done to your hair and continue treatments needed for damaged or chemically treated hair. As always check with your stylist and see what they may prescribe for your hair. You may need products that help detox the scalp or products that add protein, because the hair may need more strength and the hair fibers need to be rebuilt or restructured. Whatever your reason may be for cocktailing your products, make sure you do it per stylist and manufacturer guidelines. They would be the ones who would know what's best for anyone who wants to mix a product or two together. Cocktailing for anyone can be really adventurous and your hair will tell you whether or not it approves of your creation. So it might not be a bad idea to journal your treatment cocktail experiences. Enjoy trying the different ways to help treat your hair. The goal is finding a balance in order to achieve the desired result of the drink, I mean hair. Enjoy!

The Beauty Practice:

Check with the product company of your choice to see what they recommend when "cocktailing" their products together.

Determine the balance that's needed from these cocktailing experiences.

Journal your cocktail experiences. This will help you remember what works and what doesn't work for your hair type.

The Beauty Play #21

The Excess Heat

The Beauty Play by Play:

Blow dryers, curling irons, flat irons, crimpers, and spiral wands. What do all these tools have in common? They are all powered by heat. From wet hair to dry hair, we use some form of heat on our hair and many times the heat becomes excessive. I have a client who gets her hair done like clockwork, every two weeks and during one of her appointments with me I noticed her hair was recognizably shorter in the front. It was around her hairline. It looked as if she had cut bangs in her hair or something. I asked her what was going on and she couldn't tell me at first. She was not aware of anything that she had done different to her hair. As her appointment time continued with me she remembered what happened to the front of her hair. She said: "It's my flat iron!" She continued saying, "I have been using my flat iron just about every day on the off weeks that I don't come and see you and one morning I was rushing and did not realize my flat iron temperature had changed. It was on the highest heat setting and I didn't check it before I used it in my hair that morning. My hair felt kind of singed but I didn't really pay much attention to it, I was rushing."

Well that was easy enough, I thought. It was a combination of the excess heat of the flat iron and her rushing that was the culprit to her sudden breakage to her hair. I began to gently explain to her that she needed to back off using the flat iron so often. The hair does not need to have the flat iron or any other hot tool on the hair every day. This is called excessive use and when you use a hot tool every single day, you are bound to get results to the hair that is not favorable.

As I share with all my clients and now with you, protect your hair. It is a delicate fiber that needs to be treated as such. Apply a hair protectant to the hair before you use your heated tools. Make sure your hair is getting the right amount of moisture especially with all these high powered hair tools that are on the market. Not everyone needs to blow dry, curl, or flat iron their hair on the hottest setting. These new tools come in various temperature control settings, take time to get to know your equipment. Do a test run on a piece of your hair (preferably underneath in the back of your hair) to test the heat setting of your choice before engaging your whole head to the excess heat. And by all means if you are in a hurry do not perform any of these services with these hot tools. You don't want my clients experience to be yours.

The Beauty Practice:

Pay attention to the settings on your hot tools.

Perform a test strand with your irons in the back of the head to make sure the desired setting is not too hot for the hair especially if you have a new tool.

Use a form of heat protectant to the hair every time you use your irons or blow dryer.

The Beauty Play #22

Keep Your Hands Out!

The Beauty Play by Play:

If I had a dollar every time someone got on me for having my hands in my hair I would be rich. I just can't help it; it's soothing to play in my hair. It's like my security blanket. Even though it is soothing too me, I am really causing harm to my hair. Every time I put my hand in my hair or rub my scalp, I end up pulling out a few strands. Over a period of time I have caused the hair to weaken because I just can't seem to keep my hands out of my head. I know the lasting and visible effects such as: thinning, premature shedding and possibly balding it's causing and I can't seem to stop.

I know I am not the only person like this. I know there are other people just like me. Let me share with you what I do to combat this problem of many years. I make sure my hair and scalp are nice and clean. Shampooing my hair more often helps keep my hands out of my hair. I have told my younger clients for years not to let anyone touch their hair after they first get it done and it seems to work. They don't play in their hair and they don't let anyone else do it either. So I have adopted that for myself. I brush my hair with a paddle brush. This helps stimulate the scalp and get the blood flowing and it keeps my hands out of my hair. Another thing I find to be beneficial for me is I put my hair in a ponytail when it's long enough. I have noticed when my hair is pulled up it doesn't leave me room to play with my hair. These are my solutions to break the habit. It allows my hair to mend and repair itself and I am able to keep the hair on my head. My hair and scalp thank me.

The Beauty Practice:

Cleanse the hair and scalp more often.

Brush the hair with your favorite brush.

Pull it back into a ponytail (If it is long enough).

Whatever you do keep your hands off of your head!

The Beauty Play #23

The Truth

The Beauty Play by Play:

The truth about split ends. They have to be cut point blank, period. There are no ways around getting split ends and preserving them, specifically if you use blow dryers, straighteners, or curling irons. It doesn't matter if you use heat every day or if you shampoo and condition the hair once a week or more times than that. Split ends come from just day to day treatment of the hair: brushing, combing, running your fingers through your hair a hundred times a day. Splint ends are bound to come because of all the things we do to the hair.

According to Wikipedia and a host of Cosmetology Books, Trichoptilosis,("Trichoptilosis", n.d.) is the technical word for split ends. It is also my favorite technical word that I still use today with my clients when discussing split ends. I like the use of this word because it fully gets the attention of my clients when I have to tell them that I am about to trim off several inches of their hair.

I learned back in my beauty school days, there is nothing that you can do for Trichoptilosis but cut off the dead ends. There is no conditioner or treatment method that will stop the inevitable from happening. Certain products may prolong the hair cut or trim, but it will not stop it from occurring. You have to keep the hair ends trimmed in order to keep the dead ends off the hair. Trimming hair every 4-8 weeks will help keep the percentage down on how much hair will need to be removed. Staying on a schedule for hair trimming will help it to grow and it will keep the hair from being so tangled. When I wear my hair long or I am wanting more growth, I get a trim every 3 weeks. Furthermore, you will experience the smoothness of brushing or combing with amazing hair freedom. No entanglement.

The Beauty Practice:

You may prolong getting your hair cut or trimmed by various styling and conditioning methods but eventually your hair will have to be trimmed or cut.

Getting your hair ends trimmed every 4-8 weeks helps the hair to be more manageable, helps it grow and stay tangle free.

Schedule your appointment today with your stylist so your hair can be free of dead ends.

The Beauty Play #24

Please Stop

The Beauty Play by Play:

This brushing habit drives me crazy!

I know, for those of you who use a brush or a wet brush on your hair while it's wet are probably shocked to hear me say the total opposite. Hair that is wet is in more of a fragile state than when it's dry. Hair tends to stretch and shed more when it's wet than when it's dry. When you brush the hair wet, it is like abuse to your mane. You add more stress to the hair and it can potentially become weakened and cause unwanted breakage.

Using a brush on wet hair is like raking your yard. You just rake and rake until you get all the leaves up. It doesn't matter if you rake the grass up with it as long as you get through the process. The same for your hair, you rake and pull. You get a knot and just forcefully brush and pull until it's all out and the hair is nice and smooth. What about all that hair that's in the brush that doesn't have to be there?

My advice to you is to be careful. Don't cause more damage than needed when using a brush on wet hair. Try using an alternate method such as combing the hair one section at a time while using a wide tooth comb. Combs tend not to rip the hair out as much as the brush does. Applying a leave-in conditioner helps detangle the hair and makes it easier to comb wet hair.

I like to apply the leave-in conditioner in the hair and then use a wide-tooth comb. Then sometimes I might go back with a regular comb to make sure all the tangles are out before I proceed to style the hair. I know this may sound like a lot of extra steps to all my brush users but it's really not. I would rather add an extra step to combing out wet hair than brushing all my hair out. You decide. Try both ways and compare *the out comb*. Pay attention to how much hair you have come out in your comb out. Same when you are using the wet brush, check to see how much hair is actually in that brush. I know you will be surprised at what you discover.

The Beauty Practice:

Apply a leave-in conditioner before you comb out the hair.

Section and use a wide tooth comb instead of a brush.

Try both methods to determine *the out comb*.

"For me the working of hair is architecture with a human element"

-Vidal Sassoon

The Beauty Play #25

Cool Water Rinse

The Beauty Play by Play:

"I need to go home and shave my legs" says my client, after rinsing her conditioner out in cool water at the end of her shampoo service. Before I got used to her saying that, it would always baffle me and I would say why? "Because you made the hair grow back on my legs from my shave this morning, she laughed." That cool water rinse gets her every time. Finally she asked me why in the world I rinsed her hair with cold water so early in the morning? My first response is always, because I can. She just lays back in the shampoo bowl, smiles and shakes her head at me. I would later go on to explain to her the benefits of rinsing the hair in cold water, as she calls it.

First we shampoo in warm water to open up the cuticle and pull out all the oils and dirt from the hair, shampooing the hair at least 2-3 times. After we rinse the shampoo out of the hair, I add the conditioner in and rinse the hair in cool water. Rinsing the conditioner out in cool tepid water helps close the cuticle of the hair, and seals in the conditioner and leaves that hair full of shine. It's pretty amazing to see the after effects of that cool water rinse. I do this rinse to just about all my clients and once my client sees the results of the cool water rinse, they normally forget all about how cold the water is, until the next visit. The benefits speak for itself.

The Beauty Practice:

Shampoo the hair 2-3 times before you condition the hair.

Rinse the hair in as cold of a water temperature as you can stand.

Pay attention to the shine it creates on the hair after the rinse.

The Beauty Playbook #26

The Accessory Kraze

The Beauty Play by Play:

Headbands, head wraps and hair accessories are great additions to the hair. They come in all kinds of different colors, sizes and shapes. The headbands, head wraps and accessories, like barrettes, come in different materials. They work great to help keep the hair off the face or add more style to the outfit being worn. All of these hair accessories are fine until they start to do more harm than good. They can damage the hairline if worn too often (like every day). They tend to absorb the moisture and the oils around the hairline which is what leads to hair breakage, especially for those of you who play sports. The combination of the headband and the sweat drying the hair out weakens the hair. Eventually that hair will shed or break right off. Make sure you are putting the oils, moisture and strength back into the hair. Read your product labels to see which product is going to be best for your hair.

That is the same thing for our sunglasses or eye wear that we rest on top of our head. Our hair gets wrapped up into our glasses and we start to pull hair out literally one strand at a time. As time goes on, we start to notice our hair getting thinner around the hairline and it is due to the tension and pulling on the hair from the glasses. This is another one of those practical practices that we have to pay close attention to since it doesn't happen all at once.

Do your best and try really hard not to get into a routine of wearing these headbands, head wraps or head scarfs (which really smother the hair all together). This goes for your daughters in your life. Teach them early not to depend on hair accessories for everyday use. Hair accessories are just for the purpose of accessorizing your hair and complementing your outfits, not necessarily to be a permanent part of your hairstyle. Instead, get creative and try different ways to style your hair.

The Beauty Practice:

There are a few practical practices I want to leave you in regards to this head wrap and accessories kraze.

When you visibly see the hair beginning to look or feel weaker, give your hair a break from the headbands. It may be a really good idea just to stop wearing them period.

Apply a moisturizer or an oil/oil serum to help bring balance and strength back to the hair. Read your product labels to make sure you are using the correct products for the breakage that you or your daughter may be experiencing.

Do not allow the headbands, head wraps or hair scarves to be a permanent part of your hairstyle. Get creative with your hair styling. You will notice a difference.

The Beauty Play #27

Oil or Not to Oil

The Beauty Play by Play:

From generation to generation women of ethnic descent were taught to oil their scalp so the scalp didn't get dry. We were taught that this was the only way to aid our scalps and get the lubricant needed to help the hair grow and create that shine. It used to be called, "greasing the scalp." In today's times it is still a ritual that many women have passed on to their children. The question usually becomes to oil or not to oil? Truthfully, this can be answered so many ways but I will give you my top two answers I share with women who ask me this question.

For young children or anyone who may be on medication, I say oil. During the adolescent stages of life oiling the scalp aids the children who may not produce enough oil that the hair needs. For those individuals that are on medication, oiling the scalp helps replenish the nutrients the hair loses due to the different types of medicines a person may be on.

For everyone else, I say not to oil. You should be able to get the proper oils needed through your products, diet, water and exercise. There is no reason the scalp has to be oiled or greased. Oiling the scalp makes the oil glands lazy and doesn't allow the glands to work properly, potentially causing the scalp to be smothered which can open up the door to unnecessary issues.

There comes a point in time that we should stop using oil excessively so our oil glands can do what they are supposed to do and that is to naturally produce oil to feed and nourish the hair.

The Beauty Practice:

Ask yourself if your scalp really needs to be oiled?

Cut back or stop using oil excessively on the scalp.

Allow your natural oil glands to work naturally so they don't become lazy.

The Beauty Play #28

How Many Times

The Beauty Play by Play:

For years different cultures were taught to shampoo their hair every day, and in other cultures it has been taught to shampoo their hair once a week or every other week. While neither one of these ways are considered wrong, people were not taught why different cultures clean their hair more or less times. There are several things you need to take into account when deciding how often you should shampoo your hair.

For example, if you are an active person, do you work out on regular basis? Are you an athlete? Do you work out in the yard a lot? Do you perspire due to hormones or activities that would cause you to sweat? When you sweat do you sweat in your head? For these reasons you may have to shampoo your hair more often to keep your hair fresh and clean because of perspiration from your activities. On the other hand, you may have color or highlights in your hair that would need to be shampooed less. This helps to save your color from fading and to help nourish the hair from the oils that are produced from the scalp. Wearing braids or any type of hair extension may cause you to shampoo your hair less. Even while on vacation, you may decide to shampoo your hair less often.

When you answer the questions above, I believe you will be able to decide how many times are right for you to shampoo your hair per days or weeks. It is all according to your activity and style of hair that you are wearing. I would ask the same questions for the younger girls in your life. The more active they are, the more their hair should be shampooed and followed with a conditioner. You want to get as much of the salt from the sweat out of the hair as soon as possible. Try not to let the sweat dry in the hair so that it doesn't cause the hair to become dry, brittle and possibly cause unwanted breakage. This applies to swimmers as well. Do not let the chlorine or salt water dry in the hair. Wash the hair as soon after you finished swimming.

A key rule like anything else is to listen, look, and feel the hair; if it feels greasy and starts to have an unpleasant odor, it's probably a good idea to go have your hair done. If it still looks good after a week, than go another week longer. You be the judge of that.

The Beauty Practice:

Ask yourself the question: Are you active or not? Do you sweat or not? Do you have color or highlights or do you wear hair extensions?

Challenge yourself to shampoo more or less depending on your hair and scalp care needs.

After any activity that causes you to sweat, shampoo the hair as soon as possible to remove the salt from the hair so the hair does not become dry, brittle or cause unwanted breakage.

Remember to follow up with a conditioner for your hair type.

61

The Beauty Play #29

Climate to Climate

The Beauty Play by Play:

We travel from place to place and from state to state. Each state we travel to may have a different climate than we are used to. Depending on where you live and where you travel, you are bound to enter into a different climate that will affect your hair and skin. You may go from humidity to no humidity. You may go to a state that has a higher elevation which means there is less oxygen in the air. I remember visiting Colorado and having a hard time adjusting to the high altitude. Not only was it hard to breathe, my skin was a lot drier than any other state I had been before, but I had great hair days. I had to concentrate on adding more moisture to my skin than normal and didn't have to do anything to my hair.

When I travel to Florida, I know I have to prepare myself differently than I did for Colorado. I need less moisture for my skin and more moisture for my hair because of the heat in Florida. That would be true for all states. I use these two states as examples to show you the difference in the way your hair and skin are going to react. Good hair days in Colorado not so good hair days in Florida are what I have discovered.

Wherever you travel you need to know that your hair and skin is going to be affected. When you begin preparing for your travels, make sure to take into account that the items used at home may not work for you on your travels. Even for people who travel all the time, remembering what product you use or the hair style you wear in one state may not work as well in another state. Going from climate to climate may mean an adjustment in your products. You may have to change up your hairstyle for the different climates as well. My favorite advice to share with people is pay attention to what your skin and hair are trying to tell you; adjust accordingly.

The Beauty Practice:

Pack according to the climate, not only for your clothes but for your hair and skin. You may need to add more moisture (Colorado) or use less moisture (Florida). This may hold true for your hairstyle as well. You may have to change what you're doing depending on where you are traveling.

Pay attention to what your skin, hair and body are saying about the climate you are in.

Adjust accordingly to make sure you still achieve the desired results.

The Beauty Play #30

How Many Should I Use

The Beauty Play by Play:

For years the age old question has been how many styling products are safe to put in my hair at one time? Truthfully, there is no right or wrong answer to this question; there are just a recommended number of 3-4 products. Some people use as little as one product. It just depends on how *into* your hair you are. If you are a low maintenance, carefree kind of hair person then you're probably going to use fewer products. If you are you that person who likes to do a lot with styling your hair, then you are most likely going to require more products. This is why I say there is no wrong or right answer to the question.

One piece of advice I would like you to remember is the more you add the heavier the hair may become. Too many products will cause the hair to go limp, becoming too oily or heavy and could potentially make it harder to style.

I like to recommend that after you shampoo and condition the hair, you follow through with a leave-in condition or some kind of detangling product (you want to protect the hair while it is being combed out, while it's wet). Follow this with a wet-styling agent, dry the hair and finish up with a thermal protectant before you add that hot appliance to the hair. And if you are a person who likes a finishing hair spray, oil sheen or oil serum, you would do this at the final step of styling your hair.

These steps are all negotiable. You can do as you will; keep in mind what works for you and make sure you are protecting the hair from the heat. This is most important.

The Beauty Practice:

Count the number of styling products you put in your hair after you shampoo and condition it.

If you are being faced with oily or heavy hair after you dry it, ask yourself if all the products you use are necessary. Can you eliminate one or two?

Remember it is up to you. The styling products you choose to use for your hair are negotiable.

The Beauty Play #31

Going Natural

The Beauty Play by Play:

Going natural has been what I have personally thought about for many months now. I tried for several months but went back to my relaxed straight hair. What I learned in my six month stint is that the hair has to be moisturized and conditioned with a protein based conditioner. My experience is that it is a lot of work. So, needless to say, I turned back to the relaxer to maintain my hair. What I realized in my time of *Going Natural* is I needed to prepare my mind. It is a transition like any other endeavor you attempt to do. You must prepare your mind for the journey, research what you are about to get yourself into. I suggested to my clients in transition to make sure they are mentally prepared, begin to look for transitional styles, make sure they are using products to help strengthen the hair and add moisture because natural hair tends to stay on the drier side. Then decide if you are going to make the BIG CHOP, to cut all the relaxed hair off or deal with natural hair and the line of demarcation that shows the separation from the different types of textures going on in the hair.

So, now the tables are turned on me. I didn't take my own advice and then I went back to what was comfortable. Sometimes you have to get uncomfortable with things in order to get to the next level of what you are trying to achieve. Ladies, go ahead, get uncomfortable and go to the next level. When I really decide to go natural, I will make sure to prepare myself completely and not do it just because.

In short, the great thing about going natural is there really isn't a right or a wrong way to do it. This decision is strictly up to the person and how aggressive they want to be. The important thing is to be patient and give it time. Find what styles and products work for you to help you get to your desired look for your hair texture.

The Beauty Practice:

Do your homework, make sure you prepare your mind for the journey, and research what you are about to embark upon.

Decide how serious you are going to be. Will you make the big chop or will you gradually trim the previously relaxed hair off?

Be patient and give it time finding what will work best for your hair texture.

Be your own kind of beautiful!

The Beauty Play #32

Natural Hair Meets Color

The Beauty Play by Play:

There are a lot of people who believe that when your hair is in a natural state and has no relaxer or straightener in it, it is considered natural. Then you hear about the people that say natural hair comes in different forms. Well I am here to tell you the truth. Natural hair is only natural when there are no chemicals added in the hair *(natural means no chemical whatsoever)*. When your natural hair meets hair color it is no longer considered natural. Yes, your hair may still have the natural look to it but, you have technically changed the pattern of your hair. Permanent hair color relaxes the curl of the hair causing the hair texture to change and become slightly softer feeling. The hair becomes a little bit more manageable. It also causes the hair to become drier than before the color was added to the hair, therefore, you will need more moisturizing products. Color gives the hair a lot of personality, so have fun and enjoy wearing it with your chemically colored natural hair.

The Beauty Practice:

Natural hair is only natural when there are NO chemicals added to the hair.

When color is added to the natural hair, be sure to add moisturizing products to overcome dryness.

Have fun with the hair color you choose.

The Beauty Play #33

My Hair

The Beauty Play by Play:

My hair used to be so long. My hair used to be so thick. My hair used to hold a curl and now it doesn't do anything I want it to do. These are all things we have either said or what the hairdresser has heard. Recently, I overheard a conversation between a stylist and her client, and the client was complaining about the first time the stylist did her hair until now. The client was stating that she didn't understand what was going on with her hair. Every time the stylist tried to give suggestions and remind the lady of her current medical issues, she (the client) didn't want to hear that. The old phrase "we are beauticians and not magicians" still holds true today, even though we don't use the word beauticians anymore. Cosmetologists can only fix and take care of what you bring to us. Yes, it is true that the head of hair you started out with may not be the same hair you have today. We have to take into account what our current health is like, what kind of medications you may be on, your age, and all that you have done to your hair over the course of your life.

In this particular clients case, she had been growing her hair out and not getting the chemical services she normally received every 10-12 weeks because her health conditions did not permit her to. Her eating habits had changed and her medications increased. Her body was ill and so was her hair. But instead of looking at the whole picture, she only saw the glass half full.

The stylist was very professional and polite. She simply reminded the client of all her challenges she had been through in the last few months. Then the stylist reassured her that she would do her best to take care of her hair in its present state. I consider this lady blessed to have a hair stylist who actually cares. She could have had a stylist who didn't care because of the tone of the conversation. The stylist could have gotten offended. Not this person. She believes in operating in excellence and that is exactly how she handled this client.

The Beauty Practice:

Be professional, caring and excellent in everything you do.

Know your craft, skill, job, and the people you are dealing with. You don't know when you may have a similar conversation with your employer, employee or client.

DON'T GET OFFENDED! Listen to the person's needs. They may just need to vent and not need you to say anything at all, or they could just need a little reassurance that everything is going to be alright.

The Beauty Play #34

Cycles

The Beauty Play by Play:

A cycle is such an important word right now in all of our lives. We go through so many of them in one life time, from the cycle of childhood to adulthood. As women we can add to this, our monthly cycles. The older I get I notice more and more at this time of the month my hair is affected more than usual. I have realized that as my body goes through changes, so does my hair. I have gone from oily hair to extremely dry hair. My hair has gone from being pretty normal as far as the thickness is concerned to becoming thinner than it ever has been.

I've always said: one of my first things I am going to do when I get to heaven is have a talk with Eve. Seriously, we have to recognize the cycles our hair is going through. It could be the cycles of hormones, illness, stress, medicine, hair chemicals or a poor diet. Simply put, Life.

We learn to adjust our bodies as we go through different phases of life. It's important to realize these changes may also affect your hair. Along with all the other adjustments you are doing, remember you may need to alter your hair treatment, products, and maintenance care for your hair. Keep the lines of communication open with your stylist so they will be able to provide the correct service for you providing recommendations and education on ways to help you with your hair as you face the different cycles of your life.

The Beauty Practice:

Team up and communicate with your Stylist.

Beware of the condition of your health and your hair.

Consider adjusting your hair treatment, products and maintenance care according to the different cycles you may be going through.

The Beauty Play #35

Don't fuss

The Beauty Play by Play:

Before I became bored with my hair, I just did the necessary maintenance to it. I got my chemical service and my trim every 8-10 weeks. I shampooed my hair once a week, styled it, and off I went. I wouldn't use any tools on it after it was done the first time. I would just brush it thoroughly, tie it up at night, get into bed and sleep on my satin pillow case. I would wake up in the morning and untie it, brush, style and go. Truly no fussing over my hair and it was good. It was healthy. I got lots of compliments and many women asked me what do you do to your hair? I always replied with: *nothing*. I don't make a fuss over my hair. I have a routine I follow each morning and night, and I try to stay disciplined.

It was when I become bored and began to fuss, that I decided to do my hair myself. I got into trouble. Although this doesn't happen very often, when it does I suffer. Like the time I did a double color service and then did another chemical on my hair a month later. BAD MISTAKE! So I try really hard not to get bored with my hair so I don't run into this "over processing" problem. This particular time during my boredom was at the beginning of spring and I just wanted to do something different. It was a new season and I wanted to look a little different and new. Fresh for spring I thought. Those were my last famous words. I ended up having plugs out of my hair in places that were hard to cover. I had to get really creative with the way I styled my hair. I had to cover my bald spots. I wanted something different and because I went against my better judgement, the results were traumatic. I can't blame it on anyone but myself.

Now there is nothing wrong with wanting a new look, but know your limits. Because I am such a creature of habit, when I do go and do something different, I go overboard in changing it up. I get a little zealous to say the least. Do yourself a favor; don't fuss over your hair. If you are one to do so, know the limits. Know what your hair can and can't do and save yourself from all of the damage and recovery time that may follow.

The Beauty Practice:

DON'T DO IT YOURSELF!!!!!!

Know your hair's limit and make sure the new look is achievable and not going to cost you your hair.

Readjust your morning and night routine with your new look.

Maintain the health and integrity of your hair at all times.

The Beauty Play Book

Cosmetics & Skin Care Practical Practices

The Beauty Play #36

My Lip-Tips

The Beauty Play by Play:

Lipstick is by far my favorite part of cosmetics. I love my lipstick! I just can't understand why some women don't want to add this as part of their look. I have a cosmetic bag full of lipsticks and I carry it everywhere I go. I change my lip color up to three times a day. What I start off with in the morning is definitely not going to be what I end up with that evening. It's to the point where I don't start my work day off unless I have "my lips" on. Most people who know me know this one fact about me. So needless to say, I have a few tricks that work when it comes to "my lips."

I am often asked how I keep the lipstick off my teeth, and I have learned a few techniques by trial, error and by observing what works for others. My first favorite trick for keeping lipstick off the teeth is by using the old paper or Kleenex method. By placing the paper or Kleenex between your lips, pressing down and pulling the paper out of your mouth. That works really well as long as you release your lips from the Kleenex before you remove all the lipstick off your lips. My second favorite trick is to use your finger and wrap the inside of your lips around your finger and remove the excess color off that way. Another idea I think works really well is filling in the back of your bottom lip with your lip pencil that matches your lipstick. This works like a charm and it stays on longer with the liner.

As you read, you can tell I am a huge connoisseur of lipstick and enjoy all the latest and greatest colors out there. I hope this will inspire those who don't wear lipstick to at least try it. Lip gloss is ok too. The great thing about lip shades and lip gloss is that they are limitless and unrestricted. It's all about self-expression. Do what you want. Wear what you want. Anytime you want.

The Beauty Practice:

Determine what look you want to achieve with your lipsticks: bold, natural, colors that are complimentary with the clothes you are wearing.

When choosing a lip color, make sure you decide what you may want out of your lipstick. Decide if you want a moisturizing, conditioning lip color, or maybe you want some shine to the color or no shine at all, which would be considered a matte color.

Try one of the recommended techniques and discover which of the three may work for you.

Put on some lipstick and pull yourself together.

-Elizabeth Taylor

The Beauty Play #37

Lip Scrubs Work

The Beauty Play by Play:

Over the years lip scrubs have become very popular. Although lip exfoliates have received mixed reviews as to whether or not they work and if the scrubs are doing more harm than good, I am certain lip scrubs do work.

Our lips do not have a top layer of skin, known as the dermis, like the skin on our body. Our lips are made up of mucus membrane and are naturally water resistant. This is why we have to add moisture to our lips such as chapstick, Vaseline, cocoa butter, etc. . . . Lip scrubs assist in gently removing dead skin off of your lips to make the lips smooth and to help your lip color stay on longer.

If you are someone who suffers with dead skin on the lips quite often, invest in a scrub. There is nothing like having smooth lips and being able to glide your lipsticks or gloss across nice even lips. They range from store bought scrubs to homemade scrubs. Be adventurous and find one that is best suited for you. You will notice a huge difference in your lips.

Here are a few facts I have learned over the years about our kissers:

1. Licking your lips doesn't help to keep them moist. It's a temporary fix and dries the lips out even more.
2. Lips are naturally dry. You have to add moisture to the lips in order for them to be moisturized.
3. Our lips grow thinner as we get older. The collagen production decreases in the body and our lips start to lose their fullness.
4. Our lips are a muscle.
5. Like fingertips, our lips do not have identical lip impressions. No set of lips are alike.

The Beauty Practice:

Take care of your lips with good moisturizing lip balm.

Be careful not to bite or peel off the dead skin on your lips. Exfoliate them.

Stop licking your lips as a way of moisturizing your lips.

The Beauty Play #38

The Secret of the White Washcloth

The Beauty Play by Play:

As an adolescent I had really nice skin. I very seldom had breakouts. But as I became an adult I suffered from adult acne. I suffered more from the inflammation of the breakouts than the actual breakouts. I was a picker so I really stayed inflamed. I remember talking to one of my close friends at the time and she suggested changing my wash cloth for my face. I remember thinking she must be crazy if she thinks I am going to use two washcloths while showering. I had small children, there was no time for that. Eventually, I broke down and tried her suggestion, and now I won't use anything else on my face but a white wash cloth. My acne calmed down and eventually the inflammation began to soothe as well.

I have made this a practice of my shower regiment and it really works for me. Since then I have advised many of my troubled skin clients, to do the same and they say they can notice a difference as well. One of my sons has adopted this method during his shower time and he admits it has helped his face.

This is my belief behind the white wash cloth. It is dye-free and that has a lot to do with it keeping the face clean and clear. I have also noticed by using two different cloths, I don't have the fragrance from the body soap I use on my body on my face. Because my face is cleansed with fragrance free cleansers, along with the white wash cloth. And since I am a person who is very serious about the cleanliness of my face and skin care in general, the white wash cloth helps me see if I am removing all the makeup and oil off of my face. I could never see that when I used a colored wash cloth.

The Beauty Practice:

Purchase a bundle of white wash cloths just to be used on your face for facial cleansing purposes only.

Change your white cloth at least 2-3 times a week. .

For convenience use 2 white cloths. One in the shower and one on the sink. Just in case you forget to bring it into the shower. There is nothing more aggravating than jumping out of a warm shower to get what you left behind.

The Beauty Play #39

Moisture Does Matter

The Beauty Play by Play:

Were you aware lotions for the body should not be used on the face? Body lotions usually have some form of a fragrance in them. No matter how light or how strong the scent may be, you shouldn't want to put it on your face. Our face should be looked at like an artist who paints on a canvas. Before the artist paints they examine to see if the canvas needs to be primed. They do not start creating their masterpiece without the proper steps. That's the same way we should approach our skin, especially our face. We do not want to just go and put anything on it when we are in the priming stages. Just like an artist, make sure you take the time to prepare your canvas. You can start first by putting the right products on your face. Facial moisturizers contain more ingredients for the face than applying any old kind of lotion. They usually have a higher SPF in them to help protect your face from the ultra violet rays outside. They are specifically formulated for your skin type, whether you are oily, dry, combination, etc. Many facial moisturizers have products that are for individuals with skin sensitivities. While many of our body lotions advertise they do the same as the facial moisturizers, be aware the benefits are not the same. No matter which area you are moisturizing, remember moisture matters.

As you start to think about the products you use on your skin, think about the painter; you would not put the finishing spray to set your canvas before you draw your creation. Remember this would be true on your face. You must properly cleanse and moisturize the face with products that are appropriate for your skin type before you do anything else. The same for your body lotions you use. Make sure you use the correct types of lotion to get the optimum care for your skin. You will instantly feel a difference in both areas of your body.

A thought to ponder: Lotion is for the body and facial moisturizers are for the face.

The Beauty Practice:

Practice keeping the two separate. I always put on my facial moisturizer before I put on my body lotion. This way my body lotion doesn't touch my face. This is so important to me, that if I put my body lotion on first for whatever reason I will wash my hands from my body lotions and then apply my facial moisturizer. It's just that important to keep the two separate.

Take the time to read the labels of the facial products you want to use. Make sure the products you choose are going to do the job for your particular skin type.

*When in doubt, have your beauty professional help you out.

The Beauty Play #40

Sleeping in Your Make-up is a No, No.

The Beauty Play by Play:

Sleeping in your make-up ages your skin up to seven times the normal aging process. Not to mention, it makes your bed sheets dirty too. Cleansing your face before you go to bed helps to remove all the oils and makeup from your face and helps your face properly restore moisture. Just like the rest of your body when you rest, the body naturally gets replenished, rejuvenated, and refilled of its natural bodily functions. When you sleep in your makeup, your skin misses out on all the benefits that the body naturally does. Leaving makeup on your face can cause clogged pores, irritation, infection and unwanted blackheads.

I used to be that person who slept in her makeup and didn't care. I have not always stuck to this routine at night, but what honestly changed my mind was when I looked at my white down comforter one evening before getting in the bed and noticed that the comforter looked grimy. The thought immediately crossed my mind; this is what sleeping in my makeup is doing to my comforter. I can't imagine what it is really doing to my skin, night after night. The other thought I had was look at all that dead skin that I am consistently rubbing all over my face, night after night. That was enough conviction for me, and ever since then I make sure I cleanse my face every night. Now that I make it a must to cleanse my face, I don't feel right if I don't do it. Another thought that crossed my mind is do I really want to cause my skin to age prematurely? This is my other silent accountability partner as I prepare for bed at night.

I have noticed a difference in my face. It feels free and light after a long day. It feels fresh and it has a glow to it. Those benefits alone are enough for me. Not to mention my bed sheets and comforter on my side of the bed look as clean as my husband's side of the bed now.

The Beauty Practice:

Make sure you cleanse your face morning and night with a good facial wash.

Always follow up with a good facial moisturizer.

Commit to a new night time routine that includes cleansing your face before bedtime. Don't forget to moisturize afterwards. Think of this as a way to prevent premature aging.

Another helpful hint: do not use the same moisturizer you use in the morning, as you would for your night time moisturizer.

The Beauty Play #41

The Eyes Tell It

The Beauty Play by Play:

One of the first focal points people notice on a person is their eyes. Our eyes tell a lot about the person. Our eyes tell us if we have not had enough rest or if we are sick. Our eyes tell us if we are mad, surprised or unclear about something. My mother's favorite phrase was "the eyes have it or the eyes tell it." Whatever your eyes are saying, make sure they are not screaming abuse.

Our eyes and the lid areas around the eye are the most delicate area on our entire body. The eyelids are most likely the last place on our face we care for. We learn early in life how fragile this area is, but yet we abuse it. We abuse our eyes by not wearing sunglasses exposing our eyes to the sun and to the UV rays. We rub our eyes due to allergies or if a foreign particle enters the eye.   When we get sleepy we begin to rub the eyes.   When we wake up one of the first things we tend to do is rub our eyeballs. RUB, RUB, RUB is all we do to those poor eyelids, not thinking of the damage we are causing to the thinnest area on our body. And we wonder why our bottom eyelids look so puffy or dry or why we have so much "baggage" underneath them. Be gentle with your eyelids both top and bottom.

The Beauty Practice:

As you begin this new practice of taking care of the eyelids, make sure you apply your eye products carefully. You can start by not rubbing and begin to pat the product on to the area. Starting from the outside of the eye to the inner corner of the eye, using the ring or pinky finger to ensure you don't apply too much pressure to this delicate area.

Use a cool compress on your eyes in the morning and at night before going to bed. It will help with any puffiness, eye swelling or tired dry eyes. I find this to be helpful for those who wear contacts, and for those of you who have allergies. A few minutes a day help to naturally moisturize and alleviate any discomfort your eyes may be having.

To remove any make-up around the eyes, use a cotton ball with eye makeup remover on it. Close your eyes. Start underneath the brow bone and gently wipe down. If you wear mascara, you might want to let the cotton ball or cotton rounds rest a few extra seconds on the lashes to make sure you get the eyelashes clean. After you wipe from top to bottom of the eyelids, be sure to wipe underneath the eyelids from outside in. Take your time and be gentle to your eyes and be sure to invest in the right eye creams made just for this area. Eye creams also help with fine lines and wrinkles. Who doesn't want to get rid of those things anyway, right? When you use eye creams, make sure you use small amounts. You do not need to use a lot on such a small area. Plus this will help with the safety of potentially getting products in the eye.

Bottom line: take care of your eyes; you only get one set. And remember eyes tell it all. What are yours saying?

The Beauty Play #42

Wearing Unhealthy Makeup

The Beauty Play by Play:

Most women don't realize that there is such a thing as wearing unhealthy makeup. Your cosmetics are just like anything else we might use; it will go bad. The good thing is make-up takes a little longer to become harmful to our skin. A good rule to live by is if you have a particular liquid makeup you wear for example mascara, you should discard it every 3 months, especially if you open the bottle on a daily basis. And if you don't use it that often, you could keep it up to 6 months. Keeping your mascara or any other product that may have a wet consistency any longer than 6 months isn't advisable. You may set yourself up for infection from the bacteria that the product may form. As far as your powder makeup, you are safe to keep it up to 2 years. It is harder for bacteria to grow in it because of the ingredients.

Wearing unhealthy makeup should be looked at as eating rotten food. Although I may be exaggerating a bit, it still makes good sense. We would not eat rotten food that may cause us to get sick or set up food poisoning because it's harmful to the body. The same would be true for our old cosmetics. The older the makeup, the more likely it is to cause certain skin disorders, infections, or sensitivity to the skin. When make-up goes bad you begin to notice a pungent smell, or a tingling sensation when it's applied to the face. This could cause irritation, aging to the skin or cause unnecessary breakouts.

All in all make sure you are wearing new and healthy products on your face.

The Beauty Practice:

When in doubt, throw it out. Don't use old makeup!

I keep a permanent marker around to write a start date on the bottles of my products. This helps me know how long I have had the product and I don't have to guess.

Check with the manufacturer to see what their recommended time is on their products. Most lines have an allotted time on the back of the bottles that inform you of the longevity of their product. Be sure to check on that.

The Beauty Play #43

Sunscreen Protection

The Beauty Play by Play:

There are still a lot of people that don't realize the importance of wearing sunscreen. It doesn't matter how many advertisements are out on T.V., social media, magazines or in your local doctor's office, people are still in denial about using sunscreen. Most people believe sunscreen is for the fair-complected person and that's not true. Sunscreen is for *everybody,* no matter if your complexion is light, medium, or dark. The sun doesn't discriminate per your complexion. It likes us all the same. Just like the sun does not discriminate against our skin, neither does skin cancer, sun spots, nor sun poisoning. Which is why we <u>must</u> protect our skin.

Sunscreen is a protectant for your skin. It is a barrier from the sun's UV (Ultra Violet Rays) rays to the skin. Sun protectants come in many forms; there are solid sticks, lotions, sprays, cream, and it even comes in a water-resistant one. The list goes on and on.

 Sunscreen is so important for our skin, most cosmetic lines have SPF in their foundations already or they specifically have a separate bottle to purchase within their skin care line to go with the other products. Check the product line you wear to see what the SPF (sun-protection factor) levels are. I have always been taught that the higher the SPF, the greater the protection and coverage. In your quest for sunscreen make sure you look for the highest coverage.

The Beauty Practice:

When you know you're going to be outside and your skin is going to be exposed to the sun, make sure you use the proper sunscreen to help prevent sunburns. Check the labels for the SPF number.

Check to see if your foundation has an SPF in it. If not, you may need to add sunscreen before you apply your foundation. Sunscreen can be used as your moisturizer or you may add it into your moisturizer. Depending on how much moisture your skin may need.

Another thought to ponder - I like the idea of adding sunscreen in with your moisturizer; if you're in the sun nine times out of ten your skin is going to need a little more moisture. Why not get that extra dose of moisturizer on the face before heading outside.

Covering the body with long sleeves, a big brim hat, or ball cap and your sunglasses helps to protect the skin as well. There are too many tools in the beauty box not to use one of them. All you need to do is take the initiative to incorporate this one extra step before heading outside.

Protect your skin properly!

The Beauty Play #44

Acne Troubles

The Beauty Play by Play:

Acne is one of those skin disorders that can be a pain. Generally associated acne hormonal teenagers (puberty), this is not always the case. Acne can affect a person well up into their mid-to late twenties.

As a skin care specialist, I am often asked what advice I give someone with Acne. The first thing I do is remind them *I am not a Physician*. Second, I let the person know about the *Secret of the White Wash Cloth (The Beauty Play #38)* along with recommending oil free products, cleansers, moisturizers, serums and products with Salicylic Acids and even a trip to the dermatologist' office. Acne sufferers need products that go deeper than just the dermis layer of skin. They need products that provide relief and get results. I also remind my acne clients not to pick their faces which could cause further inflammation and scarring to the face. Third, I ask them to do an inventory of their daily consumption of food and water intake. When you're not eating healthy or drinking enough water this could be half of the battle for your skin. You have to take everything into account as you try to get your acne under control. So your skin can heal and your acne troubles can be gone forever.

The Beauty Practice:

Make an appointment with your dermatologist and voice your concerns to them about your acne troubles.

Pay close attention to the food and drinks you are consuming.

Check the products you are currently using on your face to see if they are recommended for your particular acne needs.

Get educated on things you can do to help your acne troubles.

SMALL TWEAKS LEAD TO BIG OUTCOMES

The Beauty Play #45

Anti-Aging the Deeper Issue

The Beauty Play by Play:

Let's face it. Aging is the deeper issue. First it's facial products for acne and then it becomes products for the wrinkles and fine lines you begin to notice. Then we begin to buy creams to help diminish the big pores on our face. We start to notice sagging so we start the hunt for the right products to help with the lack of elasticity in the face. It becomes one product after another. Our cosmetic bags and bathroom drawers seem to be swelling from all the products you have bought, trying to reverse the anti-aging process. Let's slow down and look at which products really work for this aging process. You want to purchase products that are made for this particular issue. Products that have ingredients in them such as Vitamin C and collagen. We should choose products that help improve fine lines, wrinkles and help with poor elasticity in the face.

Facial products shouldn't just sit on the dermis layer, but they should penetrate underneath the skin, to the epidermis layer. You want to see improvement in your skin within a few days. What you don't want to happen is products just sitting on your face doing nothing.

Before you purchase your facial products, look for the action words like firm, tighten, tone, strengthen, repair, restore, rejuvenate, revitalize or refresh. Specific words like this help explain what the function of a product is all about, and it will lead you to what the specific ingredients are in that particular product. This helpful idea will help to reduce the number of products you purchase.

The Beauty Practice:

Educate yourself. Read the labels and try the products that are best suited for your skin care needs.

Watch for the "action words" like firm, tighten, strengthen, repair, restore, rejuvenate, refresh, revitalize, etc.

When you have questions, always ask the professionals for their advice. Let them teach you on the products suitable for your current needs.

The Beauty Play #46

Switch It Up

The Beauty Play by Play:

It's time to switch it up. Change your facial regiment from season to season. What you used to cleanse and moisture your face with in the colder months should not be used in the warmer months. We are not as active in the winter months as we are in the warmer months. So we should be using products that have a little bit more oil and hydration to them than we would in the summer months. This helps us fight against the colder elements outside. When the weather is colder, our skin needs more, and in the summer months it may need less (unless your out in the sun a lot). We are more active and our oil glands are as active as we are on the hotter days.

My advice to you from season to season is to switch it up! I know that for my skin type that tends to stay on the oily side, I have to cleanse it once in the morning, but at night before I go to bed I may have to cleanse my face twice to make sure all that excess oil and dirt is completely removed. That's not the case in the colder months. I don't have to cleanse but once in morning and once at night. Afterwards, I may have to apply a second application of my moisturizer because my face gets drier when the temperatures get really frigid.

It's really important to know your skin and when to switch up the cleansers, moisturizers and whatever else you may incorporate in your morning and night skin care regiments. If you use masks or peels on your face, pay close attention to the skin types they should be used for and what time of the year they should be used. It is up to your discretion more so than the manufacturer. It's trial by error in this case. I like to keep it simple. I know that my mask in the winter months is not going to be as beneficial for me to use as in the summer and vice versa.

Knowing when it's time to change what you're using is key. Pay attention to what your skin is telling you, what it needs and when its time switch it up!

The Beauty Practice:

Pay attention to what your skin is telling you it needs.

Learn what your face may need from season to season.

Develop a morning and night skin care regiment.

Don't be afraid to switch it up!

The Beauty Play #47

The Secret of the Satin Pillowcase

The Beauty Play by Play:

Along my journey as a professional cosmetologist and an educator, I have learned that a lot of things that work well for the hair also benefit the face. The satin pillowcase is a great example of what I mean. The satin pillowcase is as beneficial to your face as it is to your hair. It helps diminish facial creasing and wrinkles during your resting hours. When you use other fabrics on your pillows they do the opposite to the face. Other pillowcases tend to cause more breakouts; lines and wrinkles. You often look like you have been in a war when you wake up instead of waking up looking rested and refreshed. The cool, soft satin pillowcase allows your face to breath, as it glides across the pillow, allowing the moisture to stay in the face instead of being absorbed into a cotton pillowcase. You will wake up looking and feeling rested and your facial appearance will be the proof of that.

It even helps those of you who wear eyelash extensions. I highly recommend using a satin pillowcase for this purpose alone. The pillowcase helps with the longevity of wearing your lashes and it helps to keep the lashes intact. Cotton pillowcases tend to pull on the lashes and smudge them on your face causing you to have to spend time fixing your lashes the next morning.

Truthfully the benefits of the satin pillowcase are limitless.

The Beauty Practice:

As recommended from the hair side of The Beauty Play #13, Secrets of the Satin Pillowcase for the hair, I recommend the same things for the face.

Purchase your satin pillowcase today! You can find them at the local retail stores or you can order them online. You will be glad you did.

Order/purchase more than just one pillowcase. This way when you have to wash one, you can replace it with a clean one. Depending on the brand, I normally don't dry mine, but check the manufacturer's directions of that brand.

Hopefully you do, but even if you don't change your sheets that often, you should change your pillowcases at least once-twice a week.

You should start to notice a difference as you sleep on the satin pillowcase. Give it a few days before you determine if you like or dislike it. The first thing you will notice is the appearance of your skin and no lines on the face when you wake up.

The Beauty Play #48

Stop Picking

The Beauty Play by Play:

Stop picking is not just what we tell our children to do when they are aggravating one another. It is also a phrase of reference as they grow into their teenage years and begin to pick their faces. Being a picker is a condition that people have done for years. First it's picking on our siblings and then it becomes our face.

Because our skin becomes the picking target, we end up picking at every little thing: we pick into a sore and then once it heals we pick the scab. It is almost like a never ending cycle. I have realized as someone who picks and has a child who does the same thing it is because our hands have to be constantly busy. I have read and believe that it is a nervous thing. Like me, people pick because we are bored, stressed or uncomfortable and picking becomes our comfort mechanism. In many cases, we do it so much we don't realize we are picking until someone points it out to us.

Picking can become such a problem to the skin that it leaves the skin irritated, inflamed and eventually causes scabs and scars that are noticeably large areas on the face. I have known people who have had to seek medical attention because the picking gets out of hand. The way I handle it is by making sure my face is clean if I'm not wearing make-up. It's when I don't have the make-up on that I get carried away with the picking to the point where my husband says, *Stop Picking*! *Give your face,* a rest he demands. So I stop and redirect my mind to do something else and keep my hands off my face. I have to admit I am a lot better now, than I used to be. I have become very conscious of my picking and when I realize I am doing it I make myself stop. This is not an easy habit to stop, but I believe with a little conscious effort and will power we can break this habit. After all, there is only so much make-up can cover up.

The Beauty Practice:

Stop picking. Stop picking. Stop picking!

Keep your hands off your face and redirect your energy elsewhere.

If you are not the person who picks, be the one who makes those who pick aware of what they are doing unconsciously to their skin. They might not realize they are picking.

The Beauty Play #49

Clean Brushes

The Beauty Play by Play:

What's the point of cleaning your cosmetic brushes? So glad you asked. It is to help keep from contaminating your brushes and to keep your face from break-outs because of dirty, make-up brushes. When you do clean your brushes, it can also help to free them from bacteria and from excess oil that may be trapped inside of them from not properly cleansing them. This can also help you minimize the amount of breakouts you experience from day to day.

In The Beauty Play #14 on the hair side, you learned the importance of cleaning your combs and brushes. Now let me share the importance of properly cleaning your make-up brushes. I know it is again something that we (including myself) are *not* in the habit of cleaning. This to me is one dirty job. It seems as if the make-up that lives in our brushes doesn't ever come clean. You can't wash your make up brushes like you do your hair brushes. You have to get the brushes wet, then apply shampoo or cosmetic brush cleaner to the brushes and gently massage the dirt out. I do not recommend soaking them in water. You have to physically manipulate these brushes clean. Let the warm water run and cleanse the brushes that way. If you soak the brushes, they are not going to get clean; they will stay full of make-up. To get your brushes clean you will have to repeat the cleansing process until there are no traces of make-up in the brushes. This could take up to 4-5 tries to get the brushes completely make-up free depending on the type of brushes you use: synthetic or natural.

I have found that there is one major challenge when you go to drying your make-up brushes. It takes forever!! So let me advise you to only clean a few at a time. You don't want to put wet brushes on your make-up compacts and ruin them. Although it may take a couple of days for your brushes to dry, it will be worth the wait. Letting your brushes air dry helps to save the shape of the brushes and will keep them intact longer. Be careful as you cleanse not to pull your bristles out. Take your time and treat your brushes right.

The Beauty Practice:

Clean your brushes to protect your face from break-outs.

Clean only a few of your make-up brushes at a time.

Cleaning Directions:

Wet, apply shampoo or brush cleaner, rinse and repeat, until the water runs clear. Let cosmetic brushes air dry to keep the shape.

The Beauty Play #50

Benefits of a Facial

The Beauty Play by Play:

Facials are a hidden treasure that many people miss out on because they don't really understand the important benefits of a facial. I am referring to the facials that are performed by an esthetician or skin care specialist. While all facials have some benefits, there are plenty more benefits going to the trained professional to receive a facial than the one you give yourself at home. Facials that are serviced by the professional help to improve the look and health of your skin as well as allowing yourself to get a little bit of relaxation during this time. Facials are known to slow down the premature aging process, deeply cleanse and unclog your pores. Facials help hydrate the skin and help with normal functioning of the fluid balance in the skin. With the right customized facial treatment, it will help give your face a smoother texture, proper hydration, fewer breakouts and firmer skin. Facials can also relieve the body of stress and toxins.

Through the right facial service from the esthetician your facial will leave your face feeling refreshed. It will bring balance to your face and calmness to your mind, body, and spirit. You owe it to yourself to go and let the highly trained professional treat your face like royalty with one of their customized facials made with you in mind. Be sure to discuss your facial concerns at the time of your consultation and consider the recommendation of the specialist.

The Beauty Practice:

Get a facial by the professional skin care specialist.

Make sure they provide the service that you are looking for.

Discuss your facial concerns with your esthetician and consider their recommendations for your skin.

Lay back, relax and enjoy your facial!

The Beauty Play #51

Unnecessary Breakouts

The Beauty Play by Play:

It does not matter if you suffer from acne or not. Unnecessary breakouts happen on the face and I have learned what the culprit can be. Over a period of time and having teenage boys with fairly decent skin, I noticed my oldest son starting to have more and more breakouts on his face. I could not figure out what was causing it. I took him to a dermatologist, and they diagnosed it as just regular teenage acne. They prescribed medication for him to take internally and gave him topical facial products. It cleared up for a little while but as soon as he ran out of the product or the medicine the acne came right back. We did this routine off and on for about three years, until one day I made a point to watch what he does to his face consciously and unconsciously. I would watch him like I was looking through a magnifying glass. My husband began to watch him as well. After carefully watching him, we both realized what he was doing. He was constantly putting his hands on his face. He was constantly picking, rubbing and scratching. When we realized this, we began to make our son aware of what he was doing so he could break this bad habit.

Being on the journey to help my son peaked my interest. So I began to study and ask questions of my clients and make them aware that they could be the cause of unnecessary breakouts to their face. Many of them began to share with me concerns they had about their skin breaking out for no apparent reason and also about their children. Here are somethings I found out.

Most people pick their face when they are bored, nervous or stressed causing unnecessary breakouts. It then becomes a bad habit, one that is really hard to break because it is done unconsciously. What begins to happen is the face becomes oily, inflamed and left with breakouts.

Many people use their cell phones and work phones without cleaning them off. Over a period of using these devices, the oil from your face begins to build up onto the phone. Every time you use the phone without wiping it off, could be potential to cause unnecessary breakouts. This is true even when you are in front of the computer or studying sitting at a desk. The hand is either resting on the side of your face or on your forehead or chin. Check to see where your face may be affected the most.

Another interesting fact I discovered is people who work out and don't shower within the first hour after their work out can cause unnecessary breakouts. The body's pores are open and sweat is sitting on the skin. Once the body dries with the sweat still on the body, it can clog the pores and cause more unnecessary breakouts. Not only does it cause breakouts to the face, you can leave the body susceptible to breaking out on the chest or back area as well.

The Beauty Practices:

Break the habit and become aware of always having your hands on your face. Find something else to do with your hands instead of constantly irritating your face. If you know someone who does this, help them by pointing this out to them. This can be a sensitive subject to the person so make sure you do it in love not to upset or hurt the person's feelings. We want to help the person, not cause them anymore stress.

Clean off your phones and keep your hands off of your forehead, chin and off the sides of your face.

After your workout, go shower and get that sweat off your body. If you are not able to shower right away, at least rinse your face off.

The Beauty Play #52

Creepy Skin

The Beauty Play by Play:

Yes, you read it correctly. This is what our skin starts to look like between the ages of 30-50 years of age. The correct name for it is crepey skin named after the crepe paper we use for arts and crafts or for decorating for birthday parties. What I have found to be true is that the skin loses its moisture and the dermis layer starts to thin out and cause our skin to look dry, old and shriveled up. According to thedermareview.com, crepey skin is also caused by the body slowing down production of elastin and collagen, the proteins that allow the skin to stretch and contract in the body. Crepey skin is not the same as wrinkles. Wrinkles come from doing a particular motion in one area over and over age. Crepey skin actually comes from the thinning of our skin not being able to bounce back and return to its normal state. Crepey skin comes from our age, hormones, lack of moisture in that area of your body and sun damage. It can affect areas such as your face, neck, under arm area, hands, elbows and your décolletage. Crepey skin makes your skin sag or look like a dried up raisin. I think it really does make the skin look creepy.

I began to notice this was happening to me in my décolletage area but I didn't pay that close attention to it until I saw an infomercial about it. I saw actual pictures of how other woman were suffering from this skin that looks old and creepy. It caught my attention not only for me but for others that may be experiencing the same thing and just not know what to do for it or ignored it like I did. What I saw on that infomercial did not look good or sit well with me. I understand we will go through body transformations as we get older, but if there is help out there for me to educate myself on ways to combat or help fix the situation, I will do it. I will go and purchase products to help me along the way. I will tell others about it, just like I'm telling you.

So what can I do, you ask?

The Beauty Practices:

Drink more water. The onset of Crepey skin comes from lack of moisture and hydration to the skin. Let's keep that skin hydrated.

We can use topical creams and lotions to help improve the appearance of that dried up looking skin. This will help add moisture back into the skin that is thirsty for outer hydration.

You can also add a vitamin supplement to your diet to help you from the inside out.

I REGRET TAKING SUCH GOOD CARE OF MY SKIN SAID NO ONE EVER.

The Beauty Play #53

Your Skin Needs It

The Beauty Play by Play:

As I continue to mature I am finding out more and more of what our skin lacks due to age, hormones and all the other things we have to do because our skin doesn't look like it used to look 5-10 years ago. It doesn't even feel like the same skin at times. Because of these concerns about my skin, I find myself looking at products that have collagen in them. Some products specify exactly the actual amount on the bottle that says, 25% more hydrating to help with the elasticity of the skin or products that say it helps speed up the natural shedding of the dead skin. I believe it is Mother Nature's way of saying change is happening, not that it's coming. It is happening and you need to help out by incorporating some of these products to help you with your aging skin. Let me just say I am in denial! This can't be meant for me. I am reminded every time I am in front of the mirror I find out something new on my body, my face especially, that this sublime message is for me.

It is important that you use products that have both collagen and elastin to help keep our skin healthy. Giving the skin its snap back to regain its shape after repetitive stretching and expanding, like a rubber band does.

But when the skin starts to lose its shape, form, flexibility and elasticity, we have to use products that help put back in what we are not able to naturally produce. I know this is *not* what you want to hear but at least we know exactly what these words mean so we can understand what these products on the shelves are telling us. Purchase products that are going

116

to have everything you need to help your aging skin. After all our skin needs it.

The Beauty Practice:

Now that you have a better understanding of what collagen and elastin is, look for the products that advertise they help with collagen and elastin.

Make sure you are seeing actual results of the product you choose. You should see some benefits from the product before you are finished with the first bottle.

Check to see if there is a money back guarantee just in case you don't see results after the recommended time frame of the manufacturer.

Be patient and make sure you use it per the manufacturer's directions.

The Beauty Play #54

Make-up Lesson 101

The Beauty Play by Play:

There are so many ways, tricks, tips and ideas of make-up application that it can be intimidating. When I teach people how to apply make-up, I always teach as if they were building a house. You want to build your house on a solid foundation so it doesn't crack or fall apart. You don't want to add paint to dry wall in a house that is not properly primed. Surely you are not going to add shutters to a house that doesn't have proper vinyl siding or brick on it. This can be true for your make-up application. Let's take a closer look.

Keep in mind all the make-up I mention comes in a variety of colors, shades, blends, and tints. Your skin type will determine what is best for you. In the case of make-up we are going to check to see if we need to prime the face before the foundation. It is not necessary to do in everyone's application, but it does help people who tend to have oily skin, have enlarged pores or because they just want a smoother look to go with their foundation. Foundation is great for coverage; it helps even skin tones and it helps give the face color. Adding some of these steps to apply your make-up may begin to extend your application time. So it just depends on when you want to add this into your make-up routine. Although highlighting and contouring is not a must; more and more people are getting into the practice highlight and contouring of the face. It is whatever you have time for in your busy schedule.

Powder and concealer are a must! You need concealer for those dark circles under the eyes or for any breakouts you may have on your face that foundation is not going to be able to cover up. Powder helps to set your make-up. The great thing about make-up is that there are not many rules anymore. You wear what you feel. While there are guidelines that are passed down from generation to generation, you certainly have to just play and see what is comfortable for you. By playing I mean see what eye pencils and shadows look best on you. Try the palettes and the single eyeshadows. Try using a number of colors together until you get the hang of it. Make-up is a form of self-expression. You get to be in control. If you are still not very comfortable, get help. I am sure you know someone who wears cosmetics well and you admire how they *MAKE-UP* their face. Get that person to help you. You can always go to the counters at your local retail shops and get help from them. My only issue with going into those places is they intimidate people. Don't you let them do that to you! They are there to provide a service and I am positive they won't mind at all to answer any questions you may have about make-up. Just think of it as the Make-up lesson 101.

The Beauty Practice:

As you began to build your house of make-up, remember there are lots and lots of colors, shades, tints, and blends you can add to your make-up supply.

Keep your skin type in mind, try colors that you are comfortable with, and add a few new colors to your collection. Broaden your make-up horizon.

Play around with your cosmetics. The rules don't always have to apply.

Ask for help. It can be a close friend or someone at the make-up counter. Whatever you find to be comfortable with is what I recommend. The make-up experience does not have to be intimidating.

The Beauty Play #55

Nicole's 5 Minute Morning Make Over

The Beauty Play by Play:

As a teenager I had all the time in the world to put on my make-up. I would sit in my room and take my sweet time putting on "my face" as my mother would call it. It wasn't until I had children a husband and a full-time job that would stop me from taking my sweet time applying my make-up. I had to learn what parts of my make-up application were important and I had to be satisfied with that. I had more to think about than just myself. I had to come up with something that would be quick but beneficial. I had to think of the main points I needed to cover, complement and go. So I played around with this for several months until I found myself putting on the areas that concerned me and that is how I came up with my very own 5 minute morning make-over. I have always had uneven skin so I knew that concealer and foundation where going to be part of 5 minute make-over. I am a pretty pale girl so I had to make sure I had on my eyes (eyeliner that is) and blush. By this time my five minutes was narrowing down and I would finish with powder to set my application and off I would go. My favorite part of make-up is my lips, and I didn't want to spend time putting that on before I dropped my boys off at the sitters, only to wipe it off so I wouldn't get it on them as I kissed them good bye. So I would wait until I was in the car before I applied my lips. My lips are everything for me, so I made sure I banked 30 seconds of my 5 minutes for the car ride to work.

Your application may be different from mine which is just fine. Just consider what you want to achieve in the morning and go from there. There is no right or wrong; it is what works best for you in that 5 minute morning make-over.

Ready. Set. Go!

The Beauty Practice:

Decide what areas you need to cover, complement and go. This will help you begin to create your own 5 minute morning make-over.

Get a routine to help you achieve your application in 5 minutes. Again, it's what work's best for you.

Begin the new routine of your 5 minute morning make-over. Don't be too hard on yourself if you don't get it all finished within that short time. Keep practicing and you will get it.

The Beauty Play #56

Tricks from the Trade

The Beauty Play by Play:

Do you ever have days when things just don't go right? Things fall apart or break on you at the wrong time? That has happened to me more times than I care to count. On one of those crazy days I dropped my favorite blush compact and I was devastated. I didn't know what to do so, quite naturally I just pitched it right in the trash as I grumbled and complained. A few weeks later I discovered that throwing my compact away was not very wise of me. I tend to go overboard when things like this happen to me. It was a few months after I had dropped the compact and tossed it that I learned I could have saved my favorite blush compact. I am not really sure where I discovered this beauty tip; it could have been a class we did in one of my beauty school projects that one of my students learned or I could have been talking with one of my team mates (co-workers) in the salon. I just know this idea came from somewhere, and this trick of the trade works! I was reminded of this trick from one of the talk shows I was watching one day and the beauty tip they gave was how to mend your crumbling eyeshadow or blush compacts. What caught my attention was they had a big stop sign that said "stop and listen" and so quite naturally I tuned in to find out why. When they showed the crumbled compacts on the table and said we can save your compacts with this one simple tip, I immediately thought about my favorite blush compact I so disgustingly threw away. I did not stop and think! These words made me remember I knew a solution but didn't use it because I did not STOP and THINK. I just acted out of pure emotion. I know by now you are saying just tell us! When you read this it's going to blow your mind. If you have heard it before and I am reminding you of something you knew and just forgot, like I did, don't be too hard on yourself. The one ingredient that could have saved my favorite blush is... ALCOHOL, old fashion rubbing alcohol (It's ok if you want to let out a little scream right here, I did!).

All you have to do is gather the broken pieces from your compact, add a few drops into your compact, press it down with a paper towel to help absorb the excess alcohol, let it dry and like that your compact has been mended and back in action! Crazy, isn't it? Instead of me going back to the store to purchase another blush I could have gotten a few more uses out of what I could have saved of my blush, instead of giving it to the trash can. Clearly, I could have saved some money as well. You live and learn is all I can say. If there is a next time, I will make sure I stop and think before I stop and have an emotional reaction. My emotional reactions always seem to cost me. I hope this little trick of the trade helps you.

The Beauty Practice:

Stop and think before you just toss your crumbled cosmetic compact in the trash.

Recycle as much as you can. Place it back into its original compact; add a few drops of rubbing alcohol in with the broken make-up, and with a paper towel press down to remove excess alcohol. Allow the compact to completely dry before you begin to use it again.

It does not matter the percentage of alcohol, but I recommend 70% or better. The higher the percentage, the more sanitary it becomes. Sterilization as well as sanitation is first.

Think about what your options are before you make a hasty decision to get rid of your make-up. This is a great way to save it and save you money.

The Beauty Play #57

There is More At the End

The Beauty Play by Play:

I learned a great trick for getting the leftover lip gloss to come down to the end of the tube by pure accident. When our lip gloss tubes are about to run out, there is still a little bit left in the tube that you could probably get 10-12 more uses out of. It would make me so mad that I could visibly see how much lip gloss I had and could not get to it. I would give that wand a hard shove or two, knowing that was not going to do a thing. It always made me wonder why these companies made these wands in the lip gloss where we could not get out all of the lip gloss. That just drives me crazy. One day I discovered by accident that we can get most of that lip gloss out of those bottles.

One summer's day I was running a lot of errands so I left my purse in my SUV. As I jumped in and out of my vehicle several times, on one of those trips back into my truck; I reapplied my lip gloss and noticed that the lip gloss was trapped in the bottom of the bottle was in the middle of the tube. What am I saying? The heat that was inside my truck warmed up my lip gloss enough to let the remaining bit slide down in the middle of the tube making it easier to get. Now I am not advising you to leave your purse in the car or your make-up bag, but I will advise you to try this idea out. Place your lip gloss bottle upside down immersed in hot water for about 5-10 minutes. This will do the same thing as the heat from the sun did to my lip gloss. This will allow you to get a few more uses out of it and definitely help get your money's worth.

Something else I discovered is there are actual make-up wands that help to scrape out the lip gloss. I found this out while surfing the web. It is strictly up to you which idea you go with. My goal is to make you aware of the other options that are available to you. Helping you improve your beauty habits and practical practices is my ultimate goal.

The Beauty Practice:

Place your almost empty lip gloss bottle upside down in a bowl of hot water. Not boiling hot water. You don't want to take the chance of melting the plastic.

If the hot water suggestion doesn't work fast enough for you, than try the lip wands that help scrap the rest of your gloss out of the bottle.

Just remember there is more at the end of the lip gloss tube. I just want you to be able to try out one of these ideas to see if they help you like they have helped me.

The Beauty Play #58

Perfecting Foundation

The Beauty Play By Play:

Take if from a girl who has to buy two different foundations to make my own. This is what I would call a waste. It doesn't make sense that I have to literally buy two different foundations to make one. I have been doing this since I started wearing foundation. You don't know how frustrating this really can be. Even with purchasing two foundations, I still have to play with my mixture to make sure it is not too much of one and not enough of the other. This was very frustrating especially if you are not quite familiar or used to mixing your colors together. Just call me *the Foundation Mixologist*.

I like to recommend, testing the color on the face and **not** on the back of the hand to find out what foundation will match your skin, I do this because you wear the foundation on your face and not on your hand. Plus, the back of your hand is usually a different shade from your face.

Today, they have mirrors in the stores that have the light bulbs that are daylight and really do help you see the color of foundation you are testing as if you were looking outside in the natural light. If the store does not have the correct lighting, I like to advise my clients to go outside, if feasible. Check the color to see if it is going to be a good match for your skin tone and for the look you are trying to achieve. As a woman with a fair complexion, I have found that this saved me a lot of time, disappointment, and money from my selection not looking the same as it did in the store. It also saved me from looking like a pumpkin. This is how I determined that I had no choice but to purchase two different foundations. The good thing is there are enough brands on the market to help you choose the right colors. I just hope your quest in finding the right shade is better than mine has been. Keep your options open and try as many cosmetic brands as you need to find out what works for you. It really breaks my heart to see beautiful women with awful foundation blends on their faces. Nothing pains my heart more than seeing the line of demarcation on the sides of the face and around the hairline from where the foundation does not match or blend. Don't be that girl. Take time to find the correct blend for your skin tone.

The Beauty Practice:

Hopefully you don't have to be a Foundation Mixologist like I do and you can try out a few brands and find your match for your skin tone.

If feasible, go outside in the natural light and check your blend. This will save you from that awful line of demarcation on the sides of the face and around the hairline.

Have patience; it could take you several attempts to perfect your foundation and find exactly what you're looking for. Take your time to find that perfect match.

The Beauty Play #59

Changing Your Foundation

The Beauty Play by Play:

Ultimately it's your choice to wear the foundation of your liking. It doesn't matter if you wear full coverage foundation or just powder on your face. It depends what you want to cover, smooth out or blend on your face. For years I have been wearing full coverage foundation to help with my uneven tones and my visible open pores. In my mind I wanted to wear full coverage to cover all my imperfections and still give me the flawless looking skin that I always desired to have. Recently, I have learned that I don't need the full coverage like I did in my 20's and 30's. I have been wearing this heavy full coverage foundation because I wasn't willing to try anything else, until recently. I went foundation shopping, and I was convinced from the advice I took from the lady helping me, it wasn't really necessary for me to use such a heavy foundation. And if need be I could add a little concealer or color corrector to help me achieve the look I wanted. So I said, I would give it a try.

The lesson I learned in the visit to the cosmetic counter was, age does play a part when choosing the right foundation. As a teenager, you could use full coverage foundations or whatever you want because your skin is so supple and youthful and you could get away with wearing the full coverage make-up. But the older we get the more caution we want to become. Be careful not to choose a foundation that may   weigh your face down and pronounce your unwanted lines and wrinkles.

I am a creature of habit and at times, change is a bit difficult for me. I am glad this was one time I was open to trying a different blend of foundation. I do believe there is a foundation out there for everyone now than it was in my teenage years. Be mindful to different choices and trying them out. I was glad I discovered something new. Now I don't have to mix 2 different colors together to get the color for my complexion (as I shared with you in The Beauty Play # 58).

The difference for me from my old foundation and new one is, I can barely tell I have it on. The old foundation felt like the make-up was sliding down my face, as if I were having the 12:00 melt down all day long. I could feel the heaviness from the time I applied my foundation, until I either wiped it all away or I washed it off. Not to mention it would get on my clothes. Not anymore!

The Beauty Practice:

Decide what purpose your current foundation is doing for your skin. Do you get full coverage or not enough coverage?

Add concealer or a color corrector before applying your make-up maybe a good idea as well.

Don't be a creature of habit. Be open to new ways and ideas; if you use a full coverage try a lighter weight foundation. Light and airy is the way our foundation should feel on the face.

Adjust what you are currently wearing, especially if your age comes into play.

The Beauty Play #60

Unwanted Hair

The Beauty Play by Play:

Let's be clear. We all have it and no matter what you do to get rid of your unwanted hair it grows back. Unwanted hair is a pain in the butt. If it's not your eyebrows, it's your upper lip. If it's not the upper lip, it's the chin area. And these are just places on the face! What about the underarms and the legs? Now days it's the unwanted hair in your girl part area that needs something done other than using a shaver. Let's face it, we are just hairy people. Some more than others, but we are still hairy individuals. With the exception of the palms of our hands and the soles of our feet.

There are many options to choose from to remove unwanted hair. You may be aware of all the hair removal options that are available or just a few. Let's explore those options together. There is the good old fashioned shaving, waxing and tweezing that you can do on your own, and then there is the age old threading technique that is available and works really well. In my opinion, threading really hurts. I think it feels like tweezing, still pulling out one hair out at a time, just faster. The results look amazing if you can stand the actual process of getting it done. Other options of removing unwanted hair include electrolysis or laser hair removal which can be very expensive. I had the laser done for almost a year, and it worked really well during that time. Shortly after I stopped the service, I noticed the hair grew in other areas of my face and neck. The longer I stayed away from getting the laser service done, the more my hair eventually grew back even in the areas I initially went to have treated.

What I have learned from all my experiences of removing unwanted hair is there is not an effective way to stop hair from growing completely, unless you have a skin or scalp disorder or the hair follicles are damaged. Honestly, the best way to find what works best for you is to just test the many different options that are available. It really does depend on your budget. Once you find out what works best for you, set appointments at the salon or wherever the service is offered to help keep unwanted hair away. This helps to improve the look and feel of your skin and it keeps that unwanted hair away. I know this is a service that many of us try to do on our own, but let me recommend going to a trained professional is so much better. You will see that the end results look better and it seems to last longer.

The Beauty Practice:

If you are not accustomed to getting your unwanted hair removed, May I suggest researching and trying out the different options: shaving, waxing, tweezing, threading, electrolysis or laser hair removal.

Once you find what works best for you, add it into your budget to have the service done every two weeks or once a month, depending on how fast your hair grows.

Set an appointment at the salon to help keep that unwanted hair away. I believe that the end results look better and seem to last longer. You decide.

The Beauty Play #61

Stop and Blot

The Beauty Play by Play:

It's my opinion, one of the smartest, most brilliant inventions ever made is the blotting sheets. These particular sheets are made for oily skin or to remove excess product from the face. Blotting sheets are great to set your foundation and touch up your make-up throughout the day. The purpose of the blotting sheets is to remove only the excess oil and to help keep your make-up intact. This works so much better than wiping or blotting your make-up with your sponge. Using the blotting sheets before you use your translucent or pressed power sponge applicator helps you so you don't transfer the oil from your face to your make-up compact. I would recommend blotting before you use your pressed powder to help freshen up your make-up throughout the day.

The blotting sheets can be used on any area of the face, particularly in the areas we are prone to shine: forehead, cheeks, chins and under the eyes. You can also use the sheets for blotting the excess lip gloss or lipstick off your lips. Blotting sheets tend to work better than just using whatever you have handy. I still like to use the other examples I gave you in The Beauty Play #36.

So the next time you go to wipe your face with just any old kind of paper, napkin or even your hand, etc., *Stop and Blot* first. Do not wipe as it will lead to taking off more of your make-up than you want to take off before the day is over. To make sure you get long lasting wear out of your make-up, go and purchase a pack of blotting sheets for your face. You will be able to tell a great big difference in your make-up.

The Beauty Practice:

Stop and blot before using your sponge applicator in your translucent or pressed powder compact to get long lasting wear out of your make-up.

Do not use hard paper towels, napkins or your hand to blot your make-up. Using these items takes off more make-up than you need to.

Go and purchase your blotting sheets for your face. They are a fun beauty tool to have around.

BLEND BLEND BLEND!

The Beauty Play #62

The Beauty Blender

The Beauty Play by Play:

Many of us carry a pressed power or translucent powder compact in our cosmetic bags or in our purse to touch up our make-up during the day. We use the sponge or what some people call the beauty blend applicator that is stored inside the compact. Most of us use the sponge without thinking about how we store that sponge or how to place it back in the compact. For some people it's not important as long as it does the job it's intended to do. I believe that it is more to know than just doing the job. You should want to properly take care of the sponge inside your compact by placing the sponge applicator upside down. The actual fabric side you use for your face should be face up towards the mirror. When you place the used side down directly on your powder it will eventually cause the compact to start getting oily spots in the powder. This will ruin your compact quicker than you using it up; it can potentially cause bacteria to grow within the compact forcing you to have to throw it away due to the transference of oil from your face into the powder itself.

Repositioning your beauty blend applicator inside the compact will increase your chances to use the pressed powder up completely. The oil on the sponge will not come in contact of the powder for long periods of time. So there will be no chance of the oil being absorbed in the powder. My advice is to be proactive and purchase an extra beauty blend applicator (sponge) in advance. I always like to purchase items like make-up sponges and applicators so I have them on hand at all times. There is nothing more irritating than needing something you don't have right when you need it.

The Beauty Practice:

Reposition the beauty blend applicator in your translucent or pressed powder compact.

Purchase an extra sponge to replace the one in the compact that will eventually be too soiled to use for your compact.

Give that sponge a little more thought then getting the job done. I could save you or cost you more in the long run.

The Beauty Play #63

Shop Beauty

The Beauty Play by Play:

Have you ever thought about what is in skin care or cosmetics? Have you ever considered what it takes to make the colors, creams and powders we use daily? Let's take it a step further. Do you know what's in our products that shouldn't be? Over the years of being a training beauty consultant, I have learned that skin care and cosmetics are one of the most toxic types of products we can put on our face and body. I am referring to products such as: body lotions, deodorants, toners, sunscreens, lipsticks, perfume, body sprays, and things we use on a regular basis. I find it shocking and surprising that we as consumers read the labels of our food products but, don't do the same for our skin care. We just assume it is all good for us because of the fragrance or because of what it says on the packaging, it takes away fine lines and wrinkles. Yes, it can be what it takes away or because it smells really good but what about what's in that product. Could it be just to lure you into using that particular product brand? This is what we call marketing. What about the chemicals that are inside of that wonderful product you love so much? You have to think of this on a broader scale. Think about all that you use per day, week, month, year and over the span of your life. That is a long time to be putting toxic chemicals in your body such as parabens, lead, formaldehyde, synthetic ingredients, phthalates and the list goes on and on. These ingredients can cause serious health issues if you're not careful.

You know you love using different products on your skin and you care about what you're using on your body, or else you would not be reading this book. ☺ Make sure you are using a product from a manufacturer who discloses what's in their bottles. Product companies are in the business to sell and profit off of their goods. It is up to you the beauty consumer to become knowledgeable on your products and the ingredients inside. Through my research I have found that the companies of these products don't have to tell us everything. I have also found out that not all chemicals in your products are bad for you. Some companies are just not using what is best to go in their products. This helps them to be more cost effective. They can get more for their dollar. So, be careful and be aware of your choices for the products you want to use and choose the healthy alternative. You want the products that are absorbing into your skin in those few short seconds to be good for you and not harm your face or your body. You want the very best for your skin. After all, we only get one body to live in so make good decisions of what products to use on your body.

The Beauty Practice:

Products are very toxic and have many different types of chemicals in them good and bad; be sure to read the labels on your beauty products just like you would your food.

Become knowledgeable of the different preservatives in our products: parabens, phthalates, formaldehyde, etc. and choose the healthy alternatives.

Get the best products for your skin your money can buy.

The Beauty Play #64

Wear It Well

The Beauty Play by Play:

When I was a little girl, my mother always taught me that make-up is to enhance what you were born with. It was pretty much the same thing taught when I went to beauty school. Make-up was to be used as natural enhancer. It helps to even out skin tones, add color and brighten the overall appearance of your face. Mom's rule was make-up was not to look made up but to compliment your face. My mom was always pretty current on the latest fashion, she was very knowledgeable about make-up products and the application of makeup. She was a very stylish woman so I made sure to listen to her wisdom about how make-up was supposed to be

If I had to put my mom in a category of a style of make-up she would fit in the "naturalist" category. She had beautiful skin and she liked for her make-up to look natural not the made up look. Although she was partial to the natural look, she still was aware of all the other looks out there. She taught me that there were many different looks and a variety of make-up styles you could do and she encouraged me to try the different looks. As I began to explore make-up before any of my professional training, I learned right away that I liked the natural look of cosmetics myself. I didn't like to look completely *made up,* unless I was going out somewhere that would require it (I guess you could say, I get it from my momma).

Being a professional and a beauty connoisseur, in the beauty industry; I have learned to appreciate all styles of make-up from the dramatic to the natural look; to those wild and crazy looks. It doesn't matter if you are in the performing arts or you're just a lipstick and eyeliner kind of girl. That's what makes make-up so fun. You can use it to express yourself any kind of way you choose. Make-up is so universal, it really only matters to the one who wears it. Whatever your choice, wear it well!

The Beauty Practice:

If you don't know your make-up style yet, explore the different looks until you find what you're comfortable with.

Make-up is not to be stressful or overwhelming. It is to be expressed whichever way you choose. My mom was my first teacher into the world of make-up. Find someone you trust to help you discover make-up options for the look you want to create.

Remember make- up is universal. It is strictly up to you what style you choose.

Whatever you choose wear it well!

The Beauty Play #65

Don't Share

The Beauty Play by Play:

We have all been told for years not to drink after other people. Not to eat off the same fork as someone else. Well the same is true for our make-up and our make-up applicators.

As a make-up artist I learned early that it is not wise to let other people use your personal make-up brushes or use the same make-up sponges or mascara wands. Sharing your make-up brushes and other implements is a sure way to allow bacteria to set up in your tools and can be highly susceptible to spreading infection. This is very unsanitary to share, so don't share your tools. Don't you find it alarming what you hear on the news of all the illness and diseases? Germs that are always surfacing and no one ever thinks about the little things we easily share. All I am saying is for you to think twice before you go and use other people's applicators, lip gloss or even their chapstick. Be careful not to contaminate your mascara bottles by double dipping in one single application. If you do have to share any of these products, be sure to have the extra disposable wands for that person to use. When it comes to our beauty tools we are to be cautious, clean and sanitary. You may not have realized or even thought about this as we share things so freely. Get in the mind set for all your beauty tools not to share with other folk. Germs from others are not welcome.

146

The Beauty Practice:

Keep extra wands on hand if you know you may be caught in a situation that causes you to have to share your make-up and your make-up applicators.

Help stop the spreading of communicable disease. Don't share your beauty tools. Be wise in what you do share. The best habit to get into is not to share your stuff.

Be cautious, clean and sanitary at all times. Germs are not welcome.

The Beauty Play #66

Time is of the Essence

The Beauty Play by Play:

To all my athletes and active individuals, I cannot stress enough how important it is for you to get into the habit of cleansing your body right after your workout, after a game or practice. Your pores on your body are open from sweating which can leave your body susceptible to clogged pores, causing breakouts to form on your chest, back or face from the salt left on the body. The trick to keep this from happening is showering or washing your face directly after your physical activity. It would be great if you could fully cleanse and moisturize your skin, but I do understand that doing this may not be convenient for you. Just know time is of the essence when it comes to being proactive to keeping those unnecessary zits away.

If you are unable to cleanse your body make sure you are not going for a long period of time after your workout. This can cause you more harm than good; plus it's not good hygiene. Nobody wants to smell you after you have worked up a sweat. Try to keep a cleansing pack in your bag so you have it available for afterwards. You can put wipes or towelettes in your bag. This is a quick way to remove some of the salt off the body. This works well when you're in a pinch. Be sure you moisturize your body after that quick wipe down. You do not want the skin to become dry and flaky. Putting on a little moisture back into your skin will help the skin not feel dry or tight.

The best way for me to explain is like this: You want to take care of your skin regardless of what you're doing because it represents you. It is very easy to see who takes care of their skin and who doesn't based on the appearance of the skin. I really hope you are in the number of people who like to take care of your skin rather than those who don't care about it at all.

The Beauty Practice:

Taking care of your skin after any type of activity is just good hygiene.

Get in the habit if at all possible to cleanse your skin directly after a workout, practice or a game. Removing that sweat from the body will help keep the breakouts to a minimum.

Keep a cleansing pack or cleansing towelettes in your bag, moisturizer for your face and antibacterial soap for your body followed up by using a moisturizing body lotion.

The Beauty Play #67

Facial Products for Men

The Beauty Play by Play:

Nowadays, men are just as educated and up-to-date on the latest products for their hair and skin care and they are just as concerned about wrinkles, puffiness under the eye area, acne, and clogged or big pores on their face, just like women are. The difference is there are hundreds of facial products on the market. It can be very overwhelming to purchase something off the shelf, which is typically why some men don't care what they use. What I have discovered over time and being in a house of nothing but men, is they are not willing to spend time going and reading the labels of every bottle like women do. They just want something that doesn't smell too feminine and they don't want a lot of steps involved with the products they choose.

In my opinion, this is the very reason men's facial products were invented. The packaging is catered to them. The scent is formulated for them and most of the time they don't have a lot of steps to do. It's usually the simple one (cleanse/tone), two (moisturize), three (aftershave, body spray, or cologne) and they are done. Products geared specifically for them and their skin care needs. Taking the guess work out of what they may want to use on their face.

The Beauty Practice:

If the man in your life is not using proper products for his skin care needs, encourage him to do so. Start him out with a couple of products and then gradually increase products as needed.

Make sure they are educated on what products are best for their skin, whether it comes from you or from someone who specializes in these particular areas. Help them get on a regiment of good products.

To the men who are up to-date on the current products on the market I say, good for you! Keep on taking care of yourselves.

The Beauty Play #68

Don't Knock It Until THEY Try It

The Beauty Play by Play:

Ladies, can you believe how popular men's facial hair has become? This takes skin care for men to another level. Beards are what it's all about these days. It's unbelievable. Men who weren't interested in growing facial hair are letting it grow, and men who have beards and were just letting them grow wild are now taming and training their beards by using special *Beard Products* Products.

At first I thought these products were a sales gimmick for men. But I soon learned they are not. They have products that are formulated to help men keep the condition of the beard looking healthy and maintained. It's no longer just about the alcohol and aftershave. It's about the complete array of products for the beard down to the color spray they can use in the beard. It's not used just to cover gray hair or just to darken the hair line anymore.

I have learned through my son how wonderful these products actually are because of the way they work on his beard. The products he used soften his beard and made it easy to comb through. These products gave his beard hair control and shine. I am convinced these beard products for men have changed the whole game for men taking care of their face. If you have a man in your life who is wearing his facial hair, may I suggest getting him some of these products that are out on the market. Get him some to try it out. You will be surprised at what these products do to the condition of their beards. I was totally surprised! The new beard products out there are definitely a game changer. I guarantee if you purchase these products for them and they actually use them, you will make him one happy guy! The look alone is enough.

The Beauty Practice:

Don't knock it until they try it.

Surprise the guy in your life with some of the latest beard products; he will be happy you did!

Make sure he actually uses the products.

The Beauty Play #69

The Rules

The Beauty Play by Play:

Finding the right product is a challenge alone. Don't get so caught up on the hundreds of products that are out there. Find products that work for you and use them consistently. Get into a practical practice of using them morning and night. Make sure not to form your opinion of a product until you have used it more than twice. I like to use a product for at least one month before I decide if it is working for me, unless the product causes sensitivity to my skin for whatever reason. Only you can be the judge of what is working for your skin. Make sure you follow the directions and guidelines of the product manufacturer. It is also a good idea to look at the reviews and testimonials of consumers that have previously used the product to determine whether you should use that particular product or not. It also helps to read the reviews in case you do decide to purchase the product and you run into the same issues as someone else who may have previously used the products. Keep in mind not every product is going to be for you. Your skin will be the judge of what works and what's not working.

When it comes to the massive cosmetic and skin care lines that currently exist out there, there are no rules to what you purchase, unless you are under the supervision and care of a physician. You can buy it and try it out. Make sure to check the company's policy on returns. Some companies won't let you return open or used products. So make sure you are familiar with that store's policy. My rule is if I can't return a product, then I can't purchase the product. It's your call, just know the rules.

The Beauty Practice:

Read the testimonials and reviews before the purchase.

Be consistent. Give the product time to work.

Know the rules.

The Beauty Play #70

It's Your Face

The Beauty Play by Play:

Your face is your face. It doesn't matter how you dress it up or down. What matters is how you take care of it. What matters is if you love your skin enough to take care of it. All of this depends on how you treat your face. Do you get enough sleep? Do you add sunscreen or moisture to the face? If you don't do anything to your face, that's the result you will get. Your face won't be radiant or have that healthy glow to it. It will look exactly like the way you take care of it.

Like anything else we do in life, what we put into it is what we get out of it. Keep that same thought in mind when you are looking at your skin in the mirror. To do nothing to our skin is unacceptable, especially in today's times. There are too many treatments, products, natural solutions, and chemical peels that are on the market today for you to sit back and do nothing to help your skin or help prevent certain things from happening to your skin, like wrinkles. We don't have to sit around and let them just happen. Having dehydrated skin is another one. We don't have to just let that be. There are too many trained beauty professional and doctors that can help you with your skin conditions and your skin concerns. Water alone helps with dehydration.

Love what God has given you and add good products to the body and good nutrients and water inside the body to keep it looking and feeling good. As I have said before, we only get one body. And we only get one shot at this thing called life.

Take good care of it; as the new and improved results start to show you will be glad you did you took care of your skin. you will be glad you read this book!

Seriously, it's your face, it's your body. Take care of it to the best of your ability. There are too many good products on the market not to find what will help you look your best.

May the search begin.

The Beauty Practice:

Doing nothing for our skin is not an option. Seek advice and recommendation from the beauty professional's or doctor's if need be.

Drink lots of water. Purchase good products for the body and eat well.

Love yourself enough to do a little something to improve your skin's condition and if you are a person who does it all, congratulations to you. You are on the right road to healthy looking skin. Keep up the good work and help me with the people that don't share in our small victories. Let's share what we know to be helpful with others, so they too can celebrate in the small victories of healthy looking skin!

Conclusion

I believe in victories. I believe it is part of my self-worth. What my parents instilled in me early on in life has shaped me to the woman I am today. My ultimate goal is to do all I can to make me a better person and helping others along the way.

I leave you with this: love and take care of yourself. If you don't who else will?

You only get what you are worth if you believe you are worth it.

Nicole-The Hair Coach

Hairstylists: Wonderful people who touch more hearts than hair.

The Author...

Nicole Stromberg is a licensed cosmetologist with over 25 years' experience. She is a stylist, cosmetology educator, make-up artist, product developer, former salon owner and director of two beauty schools. She is known as Nicole- The Hair Coach, a business professional who has dedicated her entire adult life to the Beauty Industry. Through her faith in Jesus Christ, her transparency, passion and desire, Nicole is called to teach, and inspire women to discover and embrace their true identity from their God given beauty inside and out. She calls it: *"Hair Coaching With A Twist"!*

She is also the proud author of Alexandria's Light Women's Devotional and the A. Light Journal. When she is not writing, teaching her students or servicing her clients. Nicole enjoys her time with her husband Robert, two sons' Alex and Keagan, family, friends and her dog named Leelo.

Like me on Facebook @ Nicole-TheHairCoach
Visit my website: Nicole-TheHairCoach.com

Bibliography

@hairbyjenne. (2016, February 2). Hair Inspirational Quotes. Retrieved from https://www.Pinterest.com

The Skin Care Foundation (2012, May 22). "Sunscreens explained": Retrieved from http://www.skincare.org/prevention/sun-protection/sunscreen/sunscreensexplained

 2018. "Trichoptilosis", Merriam-Webster.com. Merriam-Webster, (2018, November 11).

Additional Books by, Nicole Stromberg

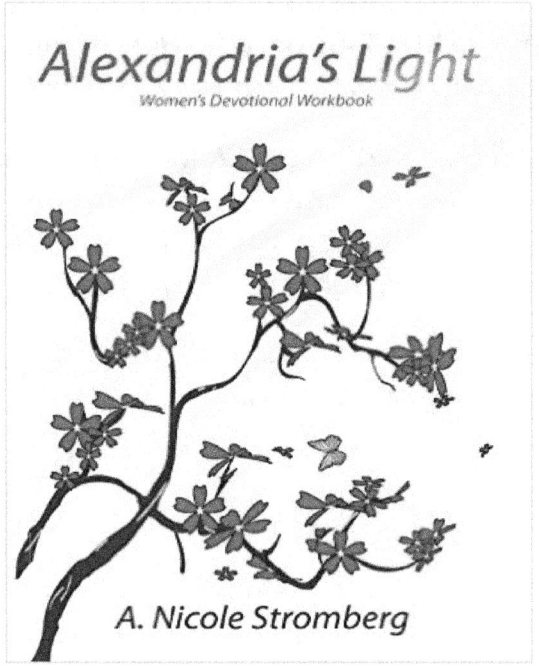

Purchase on Amazon.com

"A Light Journal" on Amazon.com